Secrets of Good-Carb/Low-Carb Living

Other Books by Sandra Woodruff

The Complete Diabetes Prevention Plan

The Good Carb Cookbook

Diabetic Dream Desserts

Light and Easy Holiday Cooking

Secrets of Fat-Free Cooking

My Doctor Says I Have a Little Diabetes

Secrets of Good-Carb/ Low-Carb Living

Sandra Woodruff

M.S., R.D., LD/N

AVERY
A MEMBER OF PENGUIN GROUP (USA) INC.
NEW YORK

Neither the publisher nor the author is engaged in rendering professional advice or services to the individual reader. The ideas, procedures, and suggestions contained in this book are not intended as a substitute for consulting with your physician. All matters regarding health require medical supervision. Neither the author nor the publisher shall be liable or responsible for any loss, injury, or damage allegedly arising from any information or suggestion in this book. The opinions expressed in this book represent the personal views of the author and not of the publisher.

The recipes contained in this book are to be followed exactly as written. Neither the publisher nor the author is responsible for your specific health or allergy needs that may require medical supervision, or for any adverse reactions to the recipes contained in this book.

Most Avery books are available at special quantity discounts for bulk purchase for sales promotions, premiums, fund-raising, and educational needs. Special books or book excerpts also can be created to fit specific needs. For details, write Penguin Group (USA) Inc. Special Markets, 375 Hudson Street, New York, NY 10014.

a member of
Penguin Group (USA) Inc.
375 Hudson Street
New York, NY 10014
www.penguin.com

Library of Congress Cataloging-in-Publication Data

Woodruff, Sandra L.
Secrets of good-carb/low-carb living / Sandra Woodruff.
p. cm.
Includes bibliographical references and index.
ISBN 1-58333-195-6
1. Low-carbohydrate diet.   2. Low-carbohydrate diet—Recipes.
3. Carbohydrates in human nutrition.   I. Title.
RM237.73.W66 2004   2004040979
613.2'83—dc22

Printed in the United States of America
1   3   5   7   9   10   8   6   4   2

This book is printed on acid-free paper. ∞

Book design by Lovedog Studio

Contents

Part II: Recipes for Carb-Conscious Living

Preface

As a practicing dietitian and nutritionist, the most frequently asked questions I have encountered over the past few years are about low-carb diets. "Are they safe?" "Do they really work?" and "Is a low-carb diet right for me?" are on many people's minds. To add to the mix, people are confused about the pros and cons of "low-carb" versus "good-carb" approaches to eating. This is why *Secrets of Good-Carb/Low-Carb Living* was written.

Secrets of Good-Carb/Low-Carb Living expands on and complements my previous work, *The Good Carb Cookbook: Secrets of Eating Low on the Glycemic Index*. *Secrets* blends the best of both worlds—beginning with a smart, low-carb plan for those of you who want a quick start to your weight-loss and health-improvement goals. *Secrets* then helps you transition to a reduced-carb/good-carb eating plan that is suited for continued weight loss and then weight maintenance. But first and foremost, this book emphasizes making choices that will help you feel your best and achieve many years of excellent health.

As you will see, one diet does not fit all. It's critical to develop a personalized eating plan geared to long-term success. The goal of this book is to help you do just that.

Acknowledgments

I am grateful for the guidance offered by the team of professionals at Penguin Group, whose input at every stage of development has made this book possible. Special thanks go to John Duff for providing the opportunity to produce this book, and to my editor, Dara Stewart, whose ongoing support, excellent suggestions, and attention to detail are truly appreciated.

A big thanks also goes to my husband, Tom, and to my friends and family members for their long-term support and encouragement. And last, but not least, I would like to express gratitude to the many clients, colleagues, and readers whose ideas, suggestions, and questions have been a constant source of inspiration.

Introduction

Low-carb diets have been in and out of fashion for decades. But until very recently, little scientific research was available to support their effectiveness. All that is beginning to change. New studies are proving that low-carb diets *do* produce better weight-loss results than conventional high-carb, so-called "balanced" diets. A lower-carb lifestyle can also be instrumental in controlling type 2 diabetes as well as prediabetes and insulin resistance syndrome—conditions that are often made worse by low-fat, high-carb diets. These discoveries are changing the way the medical establishment views low-carb diets. No longer thought of as just a "fad diet," low-carb eating is rapidly becoming a way of life for people everywhere.

Though low-carb diets show great promise for facilitating weight loss and correcting a number of health problems, many people find them tough to live with long-term. Indeed, some low-carb regimens are highly restrictive and downright boring. Others entail tedious calculations and meticulous counting of carbohydrates. And some low-carb diets are dangerously low in important nutrients and fiber, and are loaded with harmful saturated fats. Fortunately, low-carb living does not have to be difficult, nor do you have to sacrifice your health in the process.

Secrets of Good-Carb/Low-Carb Living begins by presenting the latest discoveries about low-carb diets and highlights the benefits of carb-conscious living. You will learn the pros and cons of various low-carb diet approaches and see that all low-carb diets are not created equal. But perhaps most important, you will discover why one diet does not fit all.

When it's time to put principles into practice, *Secrets of Good-Carb/Low-Carb Living* helps you do just that, with two different plans for losing weight the lower-carb way. In a hurry to get started? Then kick-start your program with the Low-Carb Quick Start Plan. If you prefer a more moderate approach, you can simply adopt the Good-Carb Life Plan to produce steady weight loss without making drastic dietary changes.

Which are the best foods for your lower-carb lifestyle? *Secrets* helps you navigate the confusing maze of low-carb foods that have flooded the marketplace, and separates hope from hype. You will also find a wealth of tips for meal planning, cooking, dining out, grocery shopping, and dealing with a variety of special situations.

The remainder of the book provides more than 160 user-friendly recipes that will make lower-carb living both easy and immensely enjoyable. Emphasis is placed on lean proteins, healthful fats, and unprocessed "good" carbs. Many of these recipes are compatible with other lower-carb eating plans such as Sugar Busters, The Zone, Atkins for Life, and the South Beach Diet. *Secrets* also includes some healthy moderate-carb recipes for sandwiches, pasta, and desserts, which can be worked into a weight-maintenance plan, or allow for those times when you want to indulge, but in a more healthful way. A complete nutrition analysis accompanies each recipe so you know exactly what you are getting, enabling you to plan meals that meet your nutrition goals.

As you will see, you have tremendous power to take control of your weight and your health. The information presented in this book can be instrumental in helping you make the right choices. It is my hope that *Secrets of Good-Carb/Low-Carb Living* can help you adopt a simple, practical, and healthful program that you can enjoy for years to come.

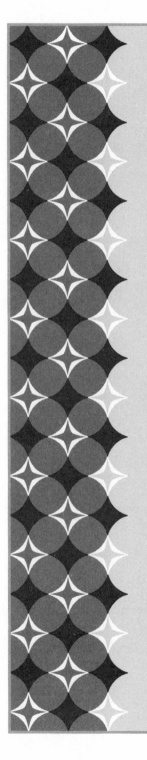

Part I

Benefits of Low-Carb Living

1.

Taking a New Look at Low-Carb Diets

In recent years, it has become abundantly clear that high-carbohydrate diets are not for everyone. Obesity, insulin resistance, and diabetes are among the biggest epidemics of our time. And cardiovascular disease remains the number-one killer of Americans. For many people, a diet too high in carbohydrate is a large part of the problem. The reason? Too much carbohydrate (especially the wrong kinds of carbohydrate) can actually make matters worse by raising blood insulin levels, triggering hunger, adversely affecting cholesterol levels, and leading to a myriad of health problems. This knowledge has led many people to take a new look at low-carbohydrate diets.

What are the principles upon which low-carb diets are based? And why are they working for so many people who have previously failed at conventional low-fat, high-carb diets? This chapter looks at the rationale behind low-carb diets and introduces the benefits of good-carb/low-carb living. The following chapters will help you devise a healthful and satisfying carb-conscious eating plan that you can enjoy for years to come.

THE THEORY BEHIND
LOW-CARB DIETS

Why do low-carb diets make sense? The rationale is really quite simple. Carbohydrates as we know them did not exist for most of history. Humans evolved eating foods that were very different from those that are available today. For instance, in the Paleolithic era, some 40,000 years ago, people subsisted on wild game, fish, and native plant foods. The only carbohydrate foods that were available were the roots, berries, and other wild plants that people foraged for. These foods were low in calories and packed with fiber and nutrients. They were also digested and absorbed slowly, providing a sustained slow-release form of energy.

With the advent of agriculture about 10,000 years ago, the human diet began a dramatic shift, as grains became staples in the diet. However, in those days, grains were eaten in their unprocessed, unrefined forms. They were left intact or coarsely crushed and made into fiber-rich porridges and dense grainy breads. Again, these foods were digested and absorbed slowly, and provided a slow-release form of energy.

Fast-forward to modern day, and a radically different picture emerges. In just the past century, our food supply has changed more than anyone could have ever imagined. Today's food supply is flooded with refined carbohydrates such as white flour, sugar, processed cereals, snack chips, and other highly processed foods—products that have no fiber and zero nutritional value, and are very quickly digested and absorbed, leading to an overproduction of insulin. These nutrient-poor, *high-glycemic-index* (see the inset "What Is the Glycemic Index?" on page 5) foods are widely available, inexpensive, heavily marketed, and served in supersize portions. Our genetic makeup was simply not designed to cope with this onslaught of refined carbohydrate. And, as you will see, the health consequences have proven to be dire.

HOW DO LOW-CARB DIETS WORK?

The benefits of a lower-carb diet are derived largely from lowering the body's insulin levels. Insulin is a hormone, secreted by the pancreas, that plays a central role in the digestion and metabolism of food. Insulin is often referred to as a "storage" hormone because it shuttles sugar and fat into cells. It also revs up the

What Is the Glycemic Index?

A theme that is repeated throughout this book is that all carbs are not created equal. One reason is their *glycemic index* (GI). The GI measures how quickly a food turns into sugar after it is eaten. High-GI foods raise blood sugar levels very quickly and tend to produce a large insulin response, the consequences of which are described later in this chapter. Refined and processed carbs like white flour, refined grains, snack foods, and sweets are the biggest offenders. A diet rich in high-GI foods has been linked to the development of obesity, heart disease, diabetes, and many other health problems. See Chapter 3 for a detailed discussion of the glycemic index.

body's fat-making machinery and inhibits fat breakdown. (If you have a weight problem, you can already see why having too much insulin around is bad news!) Some insulin is absolutely essential for life, but as you will see, an excess of this hormone can lead to a constellation of devastating health problems.

The Carbohydrate-Insulin Connection

To understand the carbohydrate-insulin connection, it helps to know a little bit about how food is digested and absorbed. When we eat, food moves from the mouth to the stomach and then to the intestines, where it is broken down into smaller particles that can be absorbed into the blood. Carbohydrates (sugars and starches) are broken down into glucose. Proteins are broken down into amino acids. Fats are dismantled into smaller fatty acids.

After a meal, glucose entering the bloodstream from digested carbohydrates triggers the pancreas to secrete insulin. Insulin then shuttles the glucose into cells, where it is burned for energy. Any glucose that is not immediately used for energy is stored in the muscles and liver for later use. Once the muscle cells and liver are filled with all the glucose they can hold, any leftover glucose is made into fat and stored in fat cells.

A couple of hours after eating, blood sugar and insulin levels begin to gradually fall. This signals the body to release some of its stored carbohydrate and fat to provide a constant supply of energy between meals and during sleep.

As you can see, we need insulin for optimal functioning. Insulin enables cells to get the glucose they need for energy. And it keeps blood glucose levels from becoming too high. Insulin also stimulates cells to take up amino acids, which are used to repair the body and create new proteins. However, a diet that is too high in carbohydrate can create an environment in which there is *too much* insulin. Herein lies the problem.

Consequences of Excess Carbs

A steady diet of overly processed, high-GI carbohydrate foods, like white bread, baked goods, snack foods, sodas, and sweets, dramatically increases the body's production of insulin. What are some of the health problems that are related to chronically elevated insulin levels?

Weight Gain

The insulin surge that occurs soon after eating processed high-GI carbs causes the digested carbohydrates to be quickly taken up by cells and stored, rather than burned for energy. As a result, blood sugar levels can become too low, too soon, leading to mild (in some cases severe) hypoglycemia. This triggers premature hunger and a roller-coaster pattern of overeating. This is also why many people feel like they are "addicted" to carbohydrates.

Cardiovascular Disease

High insulin levels promote heart disease by raising blood triglycerides (fats), lowering HDL ("good") cholesterol, contributing to increased blood pressure, promoting inflammation within the blood vessels, and increasing the likelihood that dangerous clots will form and linger in the blood.

Diabetes

A diet too high in refined and processed carbs increases the workload of the pancreas, which must secrete extra insulin to clear the excess glucose from the blood. Researchers believe that over time, the pancreas can literally wear out and lose its ability to function properly. At this point, type 2 diabetes develops.

Cancer

Diets high in refined and processed carbohydrates have been linked to cancers of the breast, prostate, colon, and pancreas. The poor nutritional quality of

The Thrifty Gene Theory

In your quest to lose weight, are your genes working against you? Quite possibly. Fat genes served our ancestors well during the hunter-gatherer period of history, when it was often "feast or famine." Indeed, researchers believe that early humans developed an innate preference for calorie-rich sugars and fats—and an ability to readily convert these calories into body fat—as a survival mechanism. This is often referred to as the "thrifty gene theory." The problem is, modern society lends itself much more to feasting than to famine. So in a world of abundance, "thrifty genes" only contribute to obesity, insulin resistance, and diabetes.

Does this mean you're powerless over your weight? Absolutely not. It has been said that "Genetics loads the gun, but environment pulls the trigger!" This is especially true when it comes to your weight. There is no doubt that genetics plays a role—and a strong family history of obesity increases the likelihood that you will have weight problems too. But gene pools change very slowly, and the explosion of obesity has occurred over just a couple of generations. This clearly shows that environment is the major contributing factor. This is good news because while we can't change our genetic makeup, we *can* manipulate our environment through positive food choices and exercise habits.

diets high in refined carbs is one reason for the increased risk. An overproduction of insulin, which stimulates the growth of cancerous cells, is another contributing factor.

Polycystic Ovary Syndrome (PCOS)

This increasingly common syndrome, which occurs in reproductive-age women, is strongly linked to an overproduction of insulin. PCOS can cause disturbances in the menstrual cycle, infertility, and a range of hormone-related disturbances.

As you can see, keeping insulin levels in check plays a crucial role in maintaining a healthy weight and preventing or treating a myriad of health disorders. Controlling your carbohydrate intake is the quickest and most effective way to lower insulin levels. It's important to realize, though, that all carbohydrates are not created equal. There's a big difference between a fresh green salad or a bowl of fresh berries and carbohydrate-laden junk foods made from white flour and sugar. Chapter 4 highlights these differences, and will help you choose the best foods to keep insulin under control *and* promote optimal health.

THE PROBLEM OF INSULIN RESISTANCE

People who are insulin resistant are especially vulnerable to the insulin-raising effects of carbohydrate. And in recent years, the number of people with this disorder has grown to epidemic proportions.

Insulin resistance is a form of carbohydrate intolerance in which people have a blunted response to the effects of insulin. If you are insulin resistant, your cells do not take up glucose efficiently, so glucose builds up in your blood. To compensate, your pancreas has to work harder to secrete enough extra insulin to usher glucose into the cells. This extra insulin allows you to maintain normal or near-normal blood sugar levels—thereby staving off type 2 diabetes. Over time, though, you could go on to develop type 2 diabetes as your pancreas becomes too exhausted to compensate any longer.

Insulin Resistance and the Metabolic Syndrome

While insulin resistance may temporarily stave off diabetes, the abnormally high concentrations of insulin circulating in the blood trigger a whole new set of problems—higher blood pressure, increased blood fats (triglycerides), lower HDL (good) cholesterol, an increased tendency for blood clots to form and linger in the blood, and increased inflammation in the blood vessels—collectively known as *the metabolic syndrome,* or *syndrome X,* all of which can triple the risk for heart disease.

How do you know if you have the metabolic syndrome? According to the National Institutes of Health, having excess fat around the belly, elevated blood triglycerides, low HDL ("good") cholesterol, high blood pressure, and elevated blood sugar are all indicators of the metabolic syndrome. Having three or more of these indicators warrants a positive diagnosis for the metabolic syndrome.

How Low-Carb Diets Can Help

Since carbohydrate is the most potent stimulator of insulin secretion, cutting back on carbs is a fast and highly effective dietary strategy for bringing insulin levels down, thereby helping to control insulin resistance and the metabolic syndrome. However, not all low-carb diets are good—and choosing a poorly planned low-carb diet can jeopardize your future health. On the other hand, cutting carbs in a smart way can not only fight insulin resistance, but also foster excellent health for many years to come. The remaining chapters in this book explain more about creating a healthy lower-carb diet.

Low-Carb Controversies

"Low-carb, high-protein diets may speed weight loss—but at what cost to your health?" critics often ask. Indeed, heart disease, cancer, kidney disease, and osteoporosis are frequently cited consequences of low-carb living. How valid are these claims? It depends largely on the *quality* of your low-carb diet. This section provides some insight about low-carb diets and health. The recipes and menus in this book will help you plan a smart carb-conscious diet that will help you lose weight *and* stay healthy for years to come.

Cardiovascular Disease

A low-carb diet based on greasy meats, high-fat cheese, butter, cream, pork rinds, and similar foods will most definitely raise your risk for cardiovascular disease by increasing your intake of artery-clogging saturated fat. Paradoxically, your cholesterol may actually drop on this type of diet while you are losing weight. This is because cholesterol typically plummets during periods of semistarvation—which is what any weight-loss diet is. Once you stop losing weight,

(continued)

you may see your cholesterol go back up. Meals high in saturated fat also cause your arteries to stiffen for several hours after eating. This forces the heart to work harder, and raises the risk for heart attack. (Since saturated fats have also been linked to the development of diabetes, Alzheimer's disease, and colon cancer, it's wise to avoid them as much as possible.)

Low-carb diets that severely restrict vegetables and fruits further raise the risk for cardiovascular disease. These foods provide a wide range of vitamins, minerals, phytochemicals, and antioxidants that help lower blood pressure, keep arteries free of deadly plaques, prevent dangerous blood clots from forming, and reduce the risk of heart attack and stroke in many other ways.

On the other hand, a low-carb diet composed of skinless poultry, seafood, lean meats, low-fat dairy products, nuts and seeds, unsaturated vegetable oils, and plenty of fiber-rich veggies and fruits can dramatically improve your cholesterol profile. Eating this way will keep harmful fats to a minimum and provide a bounty of disease-fighting nutrients that promote a healthy heart and blood vessels.

Cancer

As with heart disease, a low-carb diet may raise or lower your cancer risk—depending on your food choices. For instance, a diet that restricts vegetables and fruits will raise your cancer risk because it is woefully deficient in fiber, cancer-fighting nutrients, antioxidants, and phytochemicals. If you also eat a lot of fatty meats and dairy foods, you will make matters even worse by increasing your exposure to cancer-causing dioxins and other environmental contaminants, which concentrate in animal fats. On the other hand, a diet based on lean meats, skinless poultry, seafood, and low-fat dairy products with generous amounts of veggies and fruits is a first-line strategy for reducing cancer risk.

Kidney Disease

Eating more protein increases the workload of the kidneys, which have the job of removing protein-breakdown products from the bloodstream. However, if your kidneys are functioning normally, there appears to be no harm in consuming as much as two to three times the Recommended Dietary Allowance (RDA) for protein. In fact, new guidelines from the National Academy of Sciences Institute of Medicine state that diets providing up to 35 percent of their calories from protein are acceptable for most people.

On the other hand, if your kidneys are not functioning sufficiently, a high-protein diet can hasten their decline. The problem is that people who have kidney disease often don't know it until the disease is fairly advanced. This is why it's crucial to consult with your physician *before* making any drastic dietary changes. She or he can order a simple blood test to evaluate your kidney function.

If you are prone to kidney stones, you should also know that a high-protein diet might increase the risk of this disorder. This is because high-protein diets make the blood and urine more acidic, causing people to excrete extra calcium through their urine. Over time, this can contribute to stone formation. Restricting vegetables and fruits compounds the problem by depriving you of nutrients that counteract the excess acidity.

Osteoporosis

It is commonly believed that low-carb, high-protein diets increase the risk for osteoporosis. This is because high-protein diets make the blood more acidic. The bones react to the extra acidity by releasing some of their calcium, which acts as a buffer and neutralizes the acidity. Some of the calcium that leaches from bones is then excreted in the urine. A detrimental effect on bones is far from proven, though. In fact, some studies indicate that people who eat higher-

(continued)

protein diets (about twice the RDA) have *better* calcium retention and stronger bones than people who eat low-protein diets. This should come as no surprise when you consider that bone tissue is nearly half protein.

That said, a poorly planned low-carb diet could very well raise your risk for osteoporosis. For one thing, many low-carb diets forbid calcium-rich foods like milk and yogurt, so they are woefully deficient in calcium. Furthermore, some low-carb diets severely restrict vegetables and fruits, which makes matters even worse. Vegetables and fruits help neutralize the acidifying effects of protein, thereby sparing the body's calcium stores. Vegetables and fruits also provide a wealth of nutrients, such as vitamins C and K, magnesium, and potassium, that keep bones strong and healthy.

2.

The Low-Carb Way
to Weight Loss

Never before has there been so much debate about
what constitutes a healthy diet—especially with regard to weight loss.
Should we trim fat, calories, or both? Should we just cut back on portions? While all of these tactics are helpful, it's controlling carbohydrate
that has emerged as a frontline strategy for losing weight.

The fact is, many people who get no results with a conventional
"balanced" weight-loss diet *do* lose weight on a low-carb diet. Why do
low-carb diets work when nothing else does? This chapter looks at the
latest discoveries about low-carb diets and will get you on the road to
weight-loss success.

HOW LOW SHOULD YOU GO?

Perhaps the biggest question people have about low-carb diets is how
low should you go? Should you eliminate all carbs from your diet—or
just the "bad" ones? Confusion is at an all-time high. This why any discussion about low-carb diets must begin with a distinction between the
two main approaches to low-carb dieting—*very-low-carb* versus *reduced-*

carb. This section compares the two approaches, highlights the pros and cons of each, and will help you decide which approach is best for you. The remainder of this book will help you create a program that suits your lifestyle and personal preferences.

Very-Low-Carbohydrate Diets

When most people think of very-low-carb diets, images of bunless bacon cheeseburgers, thick juicy steaks, and piles of pork rinds come to mind. There has been a proliferation of this type of diet over the years, with the Atkins diet being the most familiar. Very-low-carb diets advocate eliminating virtually all carbs (as low as 20 grams per day, initially). They typically allow unlimited amounts of high-fat meat, cheese, cream, butter, and eggs, but only very small portions of vegetables—and no fruit, grain products, or milk at all. After a few days on this regimen, the body's carbohydrate stores become depleted, and you go into a state of *ketosis* (see "What Is Ketosis?" on page 15). This means your body is forced to burn primarily fat for energy.

Most people who have ever tried a very-low-carb diet can attest that it does promote rapid weight loss. Several factors are involved in their success. Very-low-carb diets are naturally high in protein and fat, so meals are very filling and people are not physically hungry. The ketones (by-products of fat breakdown) that begin to circulate in the blood also have an appetite-suppressant effect. And, of course, the sugary, starchy foods that most people overindulge in are completely prohibited. The end result is that people end up eating fewer calories than they normally do.

Besides preventing hunger, low-carb diets appear to have a thermogenic effect that boosts weight loss. For instance, some studies show that low-carb, high-protein diets can blunt the drop in metabolic rate that occurs with conventional weight-loss diets. The higher protein content of lower-carb diets also preserves muscle as you lose weight, which helps to maintain a strong metabolism. In addition, more calories are burned digesting and metabolizing high-protein meals, which wastes some of the calories eaten.

The Downside of Very-Low-Carb Diets

Along with the positives, there are some very real dangers associated with low-carb ketogenic diets. When you drastically cut back on carbs, your blood sugar level will plummet. For this reason, people who take medications for diabetes must work with their physician to adjust doses. If you were to continue

What Is Ketosis?

When the body is deprived of carbohydrate, it switches to burning fat for fuel. As fat breaks down at an accelerated rate, by-products called ketones are formed. Most of these ketones are burned for energy, but some are excreted through the urine, which is why people check their urine with a device called a "ketostick" to see if they are in ketosis. Some ketones are also excreted through the breath, causing the charactistic side effect of bad breath.

A highly promoted benefit to ketosis is that it has an appetite-suppressant effect, so you don't feel as hungry or care as much about food. However, there are also downsides to very-low-carb ketogenic diets, which are described below. And the goods news is that most people will find that drastically cutting carbs and going into ketosis is not necessary if you plan your diet properly. Chapter 4 presents sample menus built around lean proteins and low-glycemic "good" carbs that help suppress hunger without resorting to extreme measures.

taking the same dose of diabetes pills or insulin, you could have a serious hypoglycemic reaction. As your carbohydrate stores become depleted, you will also experience losses of sodium and water from the body—which can substantially lower your blood pressure. For this reason, people who take medications for high blood pressure must also consult with their physician about adjusting doses. If you have kidney or liver disease, you could be harmed by eating too much protein, which places an extra burden on these organs. If you are prone to gout (a condition that causes painful inflammation of the joints), a high-protein diet could cause it to flare up.

Other less serious side effects associated with very-low-carb diets include constipation—a natural result of eating so little fiber—and bad breath. In addition, some people feel weak, tired, and irritable when they cut too many carbs. Other potential side effects are headaches (the brain needs some glucose in order to function properly) and easier bruising. People who stay on this diet for too long may also notice some hair loss.

Nutritional Consequences of Very-Low-Carb Diets

The nutritional consequences of a very-low-carb diet are another cause for concern. For one thing, any diet that restricts vegetables and fruits lacks disease-fighting vitamins, minerals, antioxidants, phytochemicals, and dietary fiber. This is why very-low-carb diet programs typically recommend a plethora of nutritional supplements—which can raise your out-of-pocket costs considerably! Second, a diet high in fatty meats, butter, and cream is loaded with artery-clogging saturated fat, which may raise your risk of cardiovascular disease, colon cancer, and Alzheimer's disease down the road. (For more details, see the inset "Low-Carb Controversies" in Chapter 1.) Finally, eating high on the food chain increases your exposure to environmental toxins, which are especially concentrated in the fatty portion of meats and dairy products, potentially raising your risk for cancer.

Long-Term Prognosis

A very-low-carb diet can provide a quick start to your weight-loss efforts, but the novelty soon wears thin. After a few weeks (a few days for some people!), the thought of eating only protein and vegetables becomes intolerable and carbs start sneaking back into the diet, a phenomenon known as "carb creep." In fact, a recent study showed that after six months, most people who started out on a very-low-carb diet (less than 30 grams per day) were actually eating more than 150 grams of carb per day!

This "loosening of the rules" that happens with very–low-carb diets is evident in the weight-loss patterns of the typical dieter. The majority of weight loss occurs in the first three months. After that, weight loss slows considerably, and after six months, weight often starts creeping back up.

Can This Diet Be Saved?

There are many downsides to very-low-carb diets the way they are typically practiced—perhaps the most significant is that people simply cannot stick with them for very long. But with just a little tweaking, this diet can be greatly improved and made much more healthful and user-friendly. Chapter 4 presents a "Low-Carb Quick-Start" plan that offers quick weight-loss benefits, but with a lot less risk.

Reduced-Carbohydrate Diets

Reduced-carb diets provide about 40 percent of their calories from carbohydrate, or about 120 to 160 grams of carb per day during the weight-loss phase. The Zone, Sugar Busters, and the latter phases of the South Beach diet are examples of reduced-carb diets. Reduced-carb diets maintain the most important principle of very-low-carb regimens—protein is a key component of meals and snacks. This helps suppress appetite, preserves muscle mass, and optimizes your metabolic rate. In addition, refined carbs like white flour and sugar are discouraged, which helps keep calories under control and blood sugar and insulin levels in check. This more moderate approach also includes more "good carbs," like vegetables, milk, yogurt, fruits, and whole grains.

Since reduced-carb diets are not as drastic as very-low-carb diets, they don't cause ketosis, and they are much safer and easier to live with long-term. However, there are some practical problems with some of the reduced-carb diet plans that are promoted today. For instance, some diet plans don't emphasize lean meats, low-fat dairy products, and healthful fats, so they raise the risk for a variety of health problems. Some plans require people to eat specific food combinations in specific portions to achieve prescribed carbohydrate, fat, and protein percentages. This can be confusing and difficult to follow. Some diets offer ridiculous advice, such as warning people to avoid some healthful foods like carrots, red bell peppers, tomatoes, onions, broccoli, and zucchini because they are high in carbs compared to other vegetables or are falsely purported to cause carbohydrate cravings. And some diet plans prescribe unrealistically tiny portions.

The good news is a reduced-carb eating plan need not be tedious, overly complicated, time consuming, or skimpy with food servings. The Good-Carb Life Plan presented in Chapter 4 will help you discover simple strategies to successfully adopt a smart reduced-carb eating plan. And the tips, recipes, and menus presented throughout this book will help you build your diet around super-nutritious foods like seafood, lean meats and poultry, low-fat dairy products, plenty of vegetables and fruits, and healthful fats.

New Discoveries About Low-Carb Diets and Weight Loss

Low-carb diets have been popular for decades, but until very recently there were few good studies available on their safety or effectiveness. All that is changing as scientists around the world are comparing low-carb diets to conventional weight-loss diets. How do low-carb diets stack up?

Recent studies show that very-low-carb *and* reduced-carb diets both produce better weight loss than traditional high-carb, low-fat diets—often resulting in twice as many pounds lost. Does a very-low-carb diet produce better weight loss than a reduced-carb diet? Initial weight loss tends to be a little faster with a very-low-carb regimen, but over a period of several months, the end result is about the same. This is good news because it shows that the hunger-fighting and metabolic advantages of a low-carb, high-protein diet can be obtained without resorting to drastic measures.

The benefits of a reduced-carb diet were clearly demonstrated in a 1999 study in which a group of overweight men and women were assigned to eat all they wanted of a conventional low-fat diet or to follow a diet in which some of the dietary carbohydrate was replaced with protein. The conventional diet contained 12 percent protein and the modified diet contained 25 percent protein. After six months, both groups lost weight, but the reduced-carb, higher-protein group lost 8 pounds more than people who ate the high-carb regimen. The reason? The higher-protein group felt less hungry so they ate less food.

The *type* of weight lost on lower-carb, higher-protein diets is also consistently better than that on conventional weight-loss diets—you lose more fat and less muscle. The muscle-sparing advantage of a reduced-carb, high-protein diet was highlighted in a recent study in which researchers placed overweight women on a 1,700-calorie diet that was either high (125 grams per day) or low (68 grams per day) in protein. After ten weeks, the women lost similar amounts of weight, owing to the identical calorie counts of the diet, but women on the high-protein diet lost 2 additional pounds of body fat and retained nearly 2 more pounds of muscle than the low-protein group.

Low-carb diets also offer an advantage as far as blood sugar, cholesterol, and triglycerides go. Low-carb dieters tend to experience much better reductions in blood glucose and triglyceride levels, and greater improvements in HDL ("good") cholesterol than people on conventional high-carb, low-fat diets.

The Thermogenic Benefit of Lower-Carb Diets

Some of the calories in a meal are burned during the digestion, absorption, and utilization of that food by the body. This is called Diet-Induced Thermogenesis (DIT). DIT is a relatively small part of the calories people burn in a day, but over time it can add up. For instance, the DIT of a typical mixed meal might be 75 to 100 calories.

Fat has little effect on DIT because it requires very little work to digest, absorb, and store. In fact, less than 3 percent of fat calories get burned off through DIT. On the other hand, up to 15 percent of carbohydrate calories and 25 to 30 percent of protein calories are burned through DIT. Considering these numbers, a diet that provides ample protein, moderate amounts of carb, and not too much fat (like the eating plans presented in Chapter 4) may be best for the metabolism.

Researchers believe that the extra calories burned through DIT on higher-protein diets may help explain the greater weight loss with these diets compared with conventional weight-loss diets. In fact, a recent study found that substituting high-protein, low-fat foods like egg whites, cottage cheese, turkey, and tuna for some of the bread, cereal, and fruit in the daily diet doubled the thermogenic effect of meals.

Low-carb dieters also obtain much better improvements in insulin sensitivity. Many people are even able to reduce their dose of insulin or diabetes medications.

DO CALORIES COUNT?

Many people who adopt a low-carb diet are under the impression that calories don't count. But the truth is, they do. How do people lose weight on a low-carb diet without counting calories? The foods allowed on a lower-carb plan are more filling and satisfying, so people naturally eat less. In addition, cutting out sweets and starchy foods eliminates many of the problem foods that people typically overeat. Studies show that after a short time on a low-carb diet, most people settle into a routine of about 1,500 to 1,600 calories per day. In contrast, people who are not watching their weight may eat one and a half times to twice this amount—or even more.

If you're not losing weight on a low-carb diet, you should take a close look at what and how much you are eating. Many low-carb foods are *very* high in calories (some examples are listed below), so if you overdo it, your weight loss will stall or even stop. You might even put on a few pounds! Even healthful low-carb foods like nuts, avocadoes, and olive oil can pack on pounds if eaten in excess. Furthermore, the multitude of "low-carb" cookies, candy bars, ice cream, pasta, bread, and other foods that are now available can be very misleading. Most of these products have just as many calories as the traditional versions.

As people get closer to their goal weight, and weight loss slows, watching calories becomes even more important. Here are some examples of foods that people often eat to excess on low-carb diets.

Calorie Content of Selected Low-Carb Foods

Food	Amount	Calories
Cream	2 tablespoons	100
Cream cheese	2 tablespoons	100
Full-fat cheese	1 ounce	110
Nuts and seeds	1 cup	700 to 800
Avocadoes	½ cup cubed	120
Vegetable oils	1 tablespoon	120
Margarine and butter	1 tablespoon	100
Mayonnaise (regular)	1 tablespoon	100
Blue-cheese salad dressing	2 tablespoons	160
"Low-carb" chocolate bar	1 bar (2.8 ounces)	360
"Low-carb" muffin	2 ounce muffin	150 to 190

How Many Calories Do You Need?

There is no magic formula that can accurately predict your calorie needs. This is because calorie needs vary greatly depending on your genetics, gender, amount of lean body mass, and activity level. However, most people need somewhere in the neighborhood of 13 to 15 calories per pound to maintain their body weight. Very sedentary people may need fewer calories, while athletic people may need more.

You can estimate your calorie needs by multiplying your weight goal by 13 to 15. For instance, if your weight goal is 140 pounds, you will probably need

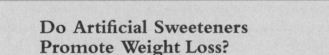

Do Artificial Sweeteners Promote Weight Loss?

The concept of using artificial sweeteners to lose weight is a simple one—by drinking a 12-ounce diet soda instead of a regular one, you could save 140 calories. Do this every day, and you could lose 14 pounds over the course of a year. But the fact is, people are using more artificial sweeteners than ever, and the rate of overweight and obesity continues to skyrocket.

What happened? Many theories abound. Some researchers believe that sweet taste, even when it contains no calories, signals cells to store carbohydrates and fats and increases appetite. Others believe that people who consume sugar-free foods make up the lost calories in other ways—take, for instance, the person who orders a burger, fries, and diet soda. Or someone may have a diet soda in the morning and compensate for it later in the day with a bag of pretzels or bigger portions at lunch.

The bottom line is that if you are serious about making dietary changes and you watch calories, artificially sweetened foods may help you lose weight by allowing you to satisfy a sweet tooth for fewer calories. If you feel like these foods stimulate your appetite, avoid them.

somewhere between 1,820 and 2,100 calories per day to maintain that weight. If you start consuming that amount of calories, you should gradually reach your goal and maintain at that level. To reach your goal faster, you can cut back a bit more, increase your activity level, or do some combination of the two. Don't cut your calories too drastically though, because you risk slowing your metabolism. In general, women should not eat less than 1,200 calories per day and men should not eat less than 1,500 calories per day.

THE BOTTOM LINE ON LOW-CARB DIETS, WEIGHT LOSS, AND HEALTH

Low-carb diets boost weight loss in a number of ways. And as more studies confirm the benefits of these diets, what was once considered just a fad is now becoming a part of mainstream medicine. A reduced-carb diet can provide results that equal those provided by a very-low-carb diet, and most people find a reduced-carb plan easier to live with long-term. In the next chapter, you will learn how to maximize the weight-loss and health benefits of your lower-carb diet by selecting healthful *low-glycemic-index* carbohydrates.

3.

Carbohydrates—
The Good, the Bad, and
the Glycemic Index

No matter what kind of eating plan you are following, you can greatly enhance your weight-loss efforts and improve your health by choosing more "good" carbs and fewer "bad" ones. What separates the good carbs from the bad? One increasingly recognized factor is the rate at which they raise blood sugar levels, or what's known as their *glycemic index*.

The glycemic index (GI) is a system that was developed in the 1980s to rank carbohydrate-containing foods based on how much they raise blood sugar levels. High-GI foods are quickly digested and absorbed, producing a quick spike in blood sugar and insulin levels. And, as discussed in Chapter 1, a diet overly rich in high-GI carbs contributes to a myriad of health problems, including obesity, cardiovascular disease, and diabetes. Low-GI foods, on the other hand, are *slowly* digested and absorbed, producing a smaller, more gradual rise in blood sugar and insulin levels, which helps protect against these disorders.

What Do the Numbers Mean?

The standard against which foods are ranked on the glycemic index is *glucose*, which has an index of 100. (Some publications use white bread as the standard, but since all dietary carbohydrate ends up as blood glucose, it makes more sense to base comparisons on glucose.)

In general, the worst carbs are foods like white bread, white rice, many breakfast cereals, and snack foods like pretzels and chips. These foods tend to have a high GI, and they provide few or no nutrients. They are also concentrated sources of carbohydrate, which intensifies their negative side effects. Sugary foods like cakes, cookies, pastries, and sodas are equally bad and are among the most concentrated sources of calories and carbohydrate available. And last but not least, baked, mashed, and French-fried potatoes contribute significantly to the glycemic load of the typical American diet. What should you eat instead? Best bets for low-GI good carbs include vegetables, fruits, legumes, unprocessed whole grains, and low-fat dairy products. Here's how some common foods stack up.

GI	*Examples*
100	Glucose
80–90	Baked potato, instant potatoes, pretzels, rice cakes, jelly beans, cornflakes, Rice Chex, and many other processed snack foods and breakfast cereals
70–80	White bread, waffles, plain bagel, corn chips, saltines, melba toast, French fries, carrots
60–70	Cream of Wheat, quick-cooking oats, whole-wheat bread (soft/airy varieties made with finely ground flour), couscous, new potatoes, table sugar, soft drinks, angel food cake, raisins, pineapple, cantaloupe
50–60	Brown rice, wild rice, popcorn, sweet potatoes, dense/coarse whole-grain breads, whole-grain

GI	Examples
50–60 (continued)	pita and tortillas, mango, banana, kiwi, sweet corn
40–50	Minimally processed cereals like old-fashioned oatmeal, oat bran, and All Bran; bulgur wheat, pasta, green peas, grapes, oranges, chocolate
30–40	Legumes, apples, apricots, pears, yogurt, milk
20–30	Barley, cherries, grapefruit, peaches, plums, soybeans
Negligible	Salad vegetables, nonstarchy vegetables such as asparagus, broccoli, cabbage, cauliflower, and green beans (A list of nonstarchy vegetables can be found in Chapter 5.)

The GI is a good starting point for choosing the best carbs, but as the latter part of this chapter will show, it's not the only thing that separates the good carbs from the bad.

Where do foods like meat, fats, and oils fit in? Since these foods are usually carbohydrate-free, they are deemed to have a GI of zero. But as you will see, that doesn't mean they can be eaten in unlimited quantities. Calories and other nutritional attributes must also be considered when planning a smart, carb-conscious diet.

THE GLYCEMIC INDEX AND YOUR WEIGHT

Perhaps the number-one reason that people are learning more about the GI and good carbs is better weight control. Indeed, mounting evidence points to low-GI, "good" carbs as being key to weight-loss success. Why? These slow-release carbs help you gain control over hunger. By producing a gradual and sustained rise in blood sugar, low-GI carbs (like vegetables, fruits, whole grains, and legumes) keep you feeling full and satisfied, and delay the return of hunger between meals.

On the other hand, high-GI carbs provide a short burst of energy that is quickly followed by hunger and a roller-coaster pattern of overeating. Many people who try conventional low-fat diets fall victim to this vicious cycle. The reason? Many foods that are mainstays of the low-fat diet—such as bagels, cereal, pretzels, snack chips, and fat-free cookies—rank high on the glycemic index. These foods are quickly digested and absorbed, causing a rapid rise in blood sugar and insulin levels. This surge of insulin puts too much of the incoming fuels into storage too soon, leaving you not enough fuel to get you through to the next meal. This is why high-GI carbs satisfy you in the short term, but soon have you coming back for more. The fact is many of the low-fat foods that people have been eating for weight loss are actually making them hungry!

The power of the glycemic index was demonstrated in a recent study in which overweight teenage boys were fed one of three different breakfasts, all with the same number of calories. The low-GI meal was a vegetable omelet and bowl of fruit, the medium-GI meal was a bowl of thick-cut oatmeal, and the high-GI meal was a bowl of instant oatmeal. Later that day, the boys were offered platters featuring a variety of foods and told to eat as much as they wanted. The boys who began their day with instant oatmeal ate nearly twice as many calories as those who got the omelet-and-fruit breakfast because they felt so much hungrier.

OTHER BENEFITS OF EATING LOW ON THE GLYCEMIC INDEX

In addition to better weight control, numerous other health benefits may be gained by lowering your glycemic load. The lower blood sugar and insulin levels that result from choosing low-GI foods can help reduce insulin resistance, improve cholesterol profiles, and fight a number of other health problems as outlined in Chapter 1. And as your blood sugar levels become more stable—instead of a series of peaks and valleys—your energy level and feelings of well-being will soar.

Can You Be Addicted to Carbohydrate?

Conventional medicine does not currently accept that people can be addicted to carbohydrate in the same sense that some people are addicted to tobacco, alcohol, or cocaine. However, people who crave carbohydrate, binge on high-carb foods, and feel powerless to curtail their intake would certainly argue with this stance. Why do so many people feel like they are addicted to carbohydrate? Here are some intriguing theories:

◆ Carbohydrates stimulate the brain to release *serotonin,* a neurotransmitter that makes you feel calm and relaxed. Researchers believe that some people indulge in sweets or starchy foods when they feel stressed or depressed as a method of self-medicating. A class of antidepressant medications known as *selective serotonin reuptake inhibitors* (SSRIs) also works by raising serotonin levels in the brain. Examples of SSRIs include Prozac, Zoloft, and Paxil. This is why carbohydrates are sometimes referred to as "Prozac on a plate."

◆ Like alcohol, sweets and other highly palatable foods stimulate the brain to release natural opiates known as beta-endorphins. Endorphins are natural painkillers and stimulate feelings of pleasure and contentment. This may be another reason why many people seek solace in food when they're feeling down. For some people, feelings of pleasure they receive from eating certain "trigger" foods is so great that they cannot stop eating them once they start, and they end up in a full-blown binge.

◆ Many people create a vicious cycle of carbohydrate craving and feelings of addiction by eating the *wrong* kinds of carbs. A diet rich in white flour, sugar, and other refined carbs can cause wide swings in blood sugar and insulin levels, leading to constant hunger and a roller-coaster pattern of overeating. Simply backing off the refined carbs and planning healthy meals featuring lean protein and fiber-rich foods can go a long way toward curbing carbohydrate cravings and restoring a feeling of normalcy.

Glycemic Index Versus Glycemic Load

The glycemic index tells you how *quickly* a carbohydrate-containing food turns into sugar, but it doesn't tell you *how much* carbohydrate is in a serving of a food. Acknowledging that both are important determinants of blood sugar and insulin levels, experts have coined a new term, *glycemic load*, which considers both the glycemic index *and* the amount of carbohydrate in a food.

Carrots, for example, have a high GI but are low in total amount of carbohydrate, unless you eat massive amounts of carrots. So compared to other sources of carbohydrate, like bread, sweets, and potatoes, the glycemic *load* of carrots is relatively low. Sugary foods (candy, sodas, cookies, etc.) and other processed carbs like white rice, snack chips, crackers, and pretzels are very high in carbohydrate *and* tend to rank high on the glycemic index. In addition, they go down easy and take up relatively little room in the stomach, so you need a large portion to feel full. These foods can dramatically raise your glycemic load.

The table on the next page provides a general idea of the glycemic load of a variety of foods. You may notice that foods tend to fall pretty much in the same order as they did when they were ranked only by their glycemic index. The main difference is that foods like carrots, which have a high GI but a low amount of carbohydrate, will be judged more favorably than if evaluated by GI alone. And concentrated-carbohydrate foods like sweets and baked goods will be judged less favorably than if evaluted by GI alone.

If you find all this talk of GI versus GL confusing, don't worry. For most people, just avoiding foods in the "high" category can dramatically improve their health outlook. Chapter 4 will put principles into practice by showing you how to use low-GI good carbs in your low- and reduced-carb meal plans.

Good Carbs—The Big Picture

Glycemic index is an important dietary concept, but realize that it's not the only thing that separates the good carbs from the bad. The reason? Just because a food has a low GI, does not necessarily mean it is good for you or that it is low in calories. Remember that carbohydrate-free foods like meats and fats have a glycemic index of essentially zero, but eat too much and you will gain weight.

Approximate Glycemic Load of Selected Foods

High	Moderate	Low	Very Low
Candy, sodas, cookies, cakes, pastries, and other sweets	Grainy breads, whole-wheat pita, whole-wheat tortillas	Milk Sugar-free yogurt Most fresh fruits	Salad vegetables Nonstarchy vegetables Nuts and seeds
White bread	Whole-grain cereals (oatmeal, bran flakes, etc.)		
White rice			
Processed breakfast cereals and cereal bars	Whole grains like barley and bulgur wheat		
Processed snack foods, like chips, prtezels, and crackers	Sweet potatoes		
	Legumes		
Mashed, baked, and French fried potatoes			

And because fat slows down the digestion of foods in the stomach, fatty foods will have a lower GI than their low-fat counterparts. Potato chips, for instance, have a GI of 54, while an unadorned baked potato has a GI of 85. This does not make the chips a healthier choice.

The high fat content of chocolate and many candy bars gives these foods a relatively low GI, even though they are high in sugar and calories. And what about nuts? They are healthful and have a low GI, but at 800 calories per cup, they are not exactly diet food! The same drawbacks can be applied to glycemic load; it's good information, but still tells you nothing about the fat, calories, or other nutritional attributes of a food.

Another problem with focusing solely on glycemic index or glycemic load is that people may needlessly shun some healthful foods, such as carrots, cantaloupe, and watermelon. These foods need not be painstakingly avoided just because they have a relatively high glycemic index. They are, after all, much lower in calories and far more nutritious than foods like white bread, sugary sodas, and junk foods, which should be the real targets for intervention. And what about potatoes—can you *never* eat one again? That would be silly. When you do eat a baked potato, make it a small portion and balance it out with low-GI foods. For instance, top a small potato with yogurt or light sour cream and have it with some grilled chicken and a garden salad.

The take-home message is that you must always temper your food choices with common sense. Use the GI as your starting point, but be sure to consider calories and other nutritional qualities of foods. Look at the big picture. Chapters 4 and 5 will help you do just this by highlighting the most healthful foods for your carb-conscious eating plan.

4.

Choose How You
Want to Lose

So far, we have looked at the benefits of controlling carbs, different approaches to low-carb diets, and the pros and cons of taking low-carb to the extreme. Now it's time to put principles into practice—with two different plans for losing weight the good-carb/low-carb way.

When approaching any weight-loss plan, it's key to individualize your program to fit your lifestyle and preferences. Everyone is different. Some people prefer a complete diet overhaul and go for quick results. Others prefer a more moderate approach. You can choose either option.

✦ Kick-start your program with the Low-Carb Quick-Start Plan and then transition into the Good-Carb Life Plan for continued weight loss and maintenance.

✦ Or simply adopt the Good-Carb Life Plan to produce steady weight loss without making drastic dietary changes.

And of course, there are acceptable variations in between. For instance, you might want to strike a compromise between the two plans by adopting the Low-Carb Quick-Start program with the addition of fruit. It's okay to experiment and find what works for you.

The Low-Carb Quick-Start Plan

The Low-Carb Quick-Start Plan is a fairly restrictive program, built around lean proteins, low-fat dairy products, nonstarchy vegetables, and healthful fats. However, it's not nearly as rigid as a ketogenic very-low-carb diet. There's no need to cut carbs so low that you go into ketosis, because most of the appetite-suppressant and metabolic advantages of a very-low-carb diet can be obtained without resorting to drastic measures.

The Low-Carb Quick-Start Plan is purely optional, but many people find that it offers some distinct advantages. Food choices are very limited, and the starchy, sugary foods that are so problematic for many people are completely taboo. This can provide a real opportunity to break some bad habits. Totally eliminating sugars and starches for a time also helps reset your taste buds so the naturally sweet flavors of foods are better appreciated. After just a few days, many people find their carbohydrate cravings begin to subside.

How long should you stay on the Quick-Start program? It's up to you—a few days, a week, or a month. Continue on the Quick-Start program as long as it's deemed safe by your physician, you feel well, and you don't feel deprived. However, to increase your chances of long-term success, you must think of the Quick-Start as just the first stage of your diet makeover. You will eventually transition to a more moderate and realistic program that you can live with long-term.

Here are the basics of the Quick-Start program. The sample menus that follow provide plenty of ideas for meal planning, and Chapter 5 provides even more information on choosing the best foods for your low-carb lifestyle. Since people rarely eat all of their meals at home, the menus also include options from a variety of different kinds of restaurants. This allows more flexibility to deal with real-life situations. Chapter 6 presents much more about dining defensively in restaurants.

Foods Permitted

+ Lean meats, skinless poultry, and seafood
+ Tofu, vegetarian meat substitutes, and legumes
+ Low-fat dairy products
+ Nonstarchy vegetables (see the list on page 62)
+ Salad vegetables

- ✦ Healthful high-fat foods like nuts, seeds, and avocadoes in moderation
- ✦ Healthful fats like olive oil, canola oil, trans-free margarine, and low-sugar salad dressings in moderation

(See Chapter 5 for more details on acceptable foods.)

General Guidelines for the Low-Carb Quick-Start Plan

- ✦ Include some protein (lean meats, poultry, seafood, dairy, or vegetarian alternatives) in meals.
- ✦ Fill at least half your plate with low-carb vegetables and/or salads at meals.
- ✦ Eat at least three times each day.
- ✦ Include some protein in snacks.

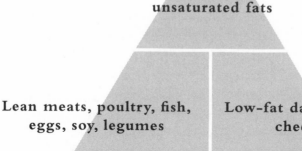

**Nuts and seeds,
unsaturated fats**

**Lean meats, poultry, fish,
eggs, soy, legumes**

**Low-fat dairy or soy milk,
cheese, yogurt**

Nonstarchy vegetables

LOW-CARB QUICK-START PYRAMID

Low-Carb Quick-Start Menus

WEEK 1	BREAKFAST	LUNCH	SNACK	DINNER
Day 1	Mushroom & Herb Omelet (page 123) 1 vegetarian sausage patty	1½ cups Lentil Soup with Italian Sausage (page 146) 3 Turkey & Artichoke Lettuce Wraps (page 224)	1 cup sugar-free chocolate milk	1½ servings Zucchini Lasagna (page 167) Mixed baby salad greens tossed with 1½ Tbsp. each light olive oil vinaigrette and reduced-fat feta cheese
Day 2	2 servings Ham & Eggs Florentine (page 131) 1 cup nonfat or low-fat milk	1 serving Gorgonzola & Walnut Chicken Salad (page 185) 1 cup reduced-sodium bean soup	8 ounces light (no added sugar) yogurt	1 serving Fish Fillets Florentine (page 177) 1 cup Green Beans with Walnuts (page 210) Garden salad with 1 Tbsp. light olive oil vinaigrette
Day 3	1 serving Cottage-Style Eggs (page 127) 2 turkey breakfast sausage links 6 ounces low-sodium tomato juice	Fast Food Restaurant: 12 ounces chili Side salad with 2 Tbsp. light ranch dressing	1 stalk celery filled with 1 Tbsp. peanut butter 1½ ounces low-fat cheese	1 serving Chicken Athenos (page 157) 1 cup Easy Baked Brussels Sprouts (page 210) Garden Salad with 1 Tbsp. Greek Isle Dressing (page 206)
Day 4	Chicken Fajita Omelet (page 125)	4 Roast Beef and Roasted Red Pepper Lettuce Wraps (page 225)	4 endive leaves, each filled with 1 Tbsp. low-fat tuna salad	4 ounces Grilled Rosemary Pork (page 174)

WEEK 1	BREAKFAST	LUNCH	SNACK	DINNER
Day 4 *(continued)*	½ small avocado, sliced 8 ounces reduced-sodium V-8	1 cup Italian Vegetable Soup (page 149)		1 cup Spring Vegetable Medley (page 214) Spinach Salad Caprese (page 196)
Day 5	Sugar-free instant breakfast drink 1 hard-boiled egg	1 serving Italian Cobb Salad (page 189) 1 cup Split Pea Soup with Bacon (page 147)	⅓ cup mixed nuts	1 serving Spicy Grouper with Peppers & Onions (page 178) 1 cup yellow squash and zucchini, sautéed in olive oil Sliced fresh tomatoes
Day 6	1 serving Microwave Egg Scramble (page 127) 1 vegetarian sausage patty 1 cup nonfat or low-fat milk	2 Portobello Pizzas (page 118) Garden salad with 2 Tbsp. light olive oil vinaigrette	2 Ham & Cheese Lettuce Wraps (page 225)	4 ounces Balsamic Braised Beef Roast (page 168) 1 cup Cauliflower with Fresh Herbs (page 212) 1 cup steamed green beans tossed with olive oil and dill
Day 7	8 ounces light (no added sugar) yogurt 1 hard-boiled egg	2 West Coast Lettuce Wraps (page 226) 1 cup reduced-sodium tomato soup	½ cup roasted sunflower seeds (measured in the shell)	Mexican Restaurant: Southwestern grilled chicken or shrimp Grilled vegetables Side of black beans

WEEK 2	BREAKFAST	LUNCH	SNACK	DINNER
Day 1	Crab & Chili Omelet (page 124) 6 ounces low-sodium V-8 juice 2 ounces turkey breakfast sausage	3 Cashew Chicken Salad Lettuce Wraps (page 226) 1 cup Summer Squash Soup (page 149)	Sugar-free instant breakfast drink	1 serving Peppercorn Pork Chops (page 172) 1 cup Savory Collard Greens (page 213) 1 cup yellow squash and onions, sautéed in olive oil
Day 2	Greek Spinach Omelet (page 124) 2 slices turkey bacon 1 cup nonfat or low-fat milk	¾ cup Sun-Dried Tomato Chicken Salad (page 191) over mixed baby salad greens 1 cup reduced-sodium lentil soup	1 piece reduced-fat string cheese ¼ cup almonds	1 serving Moussaka (page 164) 1 cup steamed green beans tossed with olive oil and dill Spinach salad with 1 Tbsp. each balsamic vinaigrette and reduced-fat feta cheese
Day 3	Zucchini & Sun-Dried Tomato Frittata (page 128) 1 cup nonfat or low-fat milk	Restaurant Salad Bar: Assorted lettuce and fresh veggies, ½ cup diced turkey or ham, ½ cup cottage cheese, 2 Tbsp. shredded cheese, 1 Tbsp. sunflower seeds, 2 Tbsp. vinaigrette dressing	½ cup pistachio nuts (measured with shells on)	1 serving Chicken Tenders with Spicy Black Beans (page 160) ½ cup Tricolored Pepper Sauté (page 216) 1 serving Guacamole Salad (page 199)
Day 4	12 ounces sugar-free chocolate milk	1½ cups Burgundy Beef Stew (page 144)	3 Ham & Cheese Skewers (page 110)	1 serving Balsamic Chicken (page 154)

WEEK 2	BREAKFAST	LUNCH	SNACK	DINNER
Day 4 (continued)	1 hard-boiled egg	Spinach Salad with 1 Tbsp. each light olive oil vinaigrette, blue cheese, and walnuts		1 cup Asparagus Amandine (page 209) 1 cup steamed baby carrots tossed with olive oil and parsley
Day 5	2 servings Asparagus, Ham, & Egg Bake (page 129) 1 cup nonfat or low-fat milk	1 serving Chef Salad with Roast Beef & Blue Cheese (page 191)	¼ cup roasted pumpkin seeds	Chinese Restaurant: Stir-fried chicken, shrimp, or tofu and vegetables Hot and sour soup
Day 6	Restaurant meal: Veggie-cheese omelet (made with fat-free egg substitute) 2 ounces Canadian bacon 6 ounces low-sodium tomato juice	1½ cups Chipotle Black Bean Chili (page 145) topped with 2 Tbsp. low-fat cheese Fresh veggies with 2 Tbsp. light ranch dressing	2 stalks celery, each filled with 1 tablespoon light veggie cream cheese	1½ servings Spaghetti Squash Casserole (page 166) Steamed broccoli and cauliflower tossed with olive oil and herbs Garden salad with 2 Tbsp. light olive oil vinaigrette dressing
Day 7	2 poached eggs 1 vegetarian sausage patty 1 cup nonfat or low-fat milk	1 cup low-fat tuna salad in a medium tomato 1 cup Cauliflower-Cheese Soup (page 151)	2 Artichoke Roll-Ups (page 116)	Steak House Restaurant: Small filet mignon Double order of grilled or sautéed veggies (instead of potato) Side salad with 2 Tbsp. light ranch dressing

Calorie Considerations

Foods on the Quick-Start Plan are very filling and satisfying, so most people will find they can get excellent results simply by eating until they are comfortably full (not stuffed) without counting calories, carbs, or fat grams. But realize that calories *do* count. (Chapter 2 provides more information on calories.) The Quick-Start menus on pages 34–37, which provide about 1,300 to 1,400 calories per day, can serve as a good starting point for planning your own personal regimen. As you plan your own meals, remember that most women should not eat less than 1,200 calories per day, and most men should not eat less than 1,500 calories. This will help you maintain a healthy metabolism as you lose weight.

MOVING FROM QUICK-START TO LIFE PLAN

After following the Low-Carb Quick-Start Plan for a period of time, most people will be ready for a more liberalized eating plan that still allows for continued weight loss. That's where the Good-Carb Life Plan comes in. At this point, you can progress your diet by gradually adding in more good carbs. For instance, have a fresh fruit cup with your morning omelet. Have a sandwich made in a whole grain pita or tortilla wrap instead of a lettuce wrap. Or add a small baked sweet potato to a meal of grilled fish and vegetables. The Good-Carb Life Plan menus in the next section will help you discover the possibilities.

THE GOOD-CARB LIFE PLAN

People who prefer a more moderate approach to changing their diet can skip the Low-Carb Quick-Start and go straight to the Good-Carb Life Plan. This plan provides about 40 percent of calories from carbohydrate, 30 percent from protein, and 30 percent from fat. Practiced consistently, this reduced-carbohydrate eating plan can produce excellent results and is much easier to live with long-term. Here are the basics of the Good-Carb Life Plan. The menus that follow provide ideas for two weeks of healthful and delicious meals.

Foods Permitted

- Lean meats, skinless poultry, and seafood
- Tofu, vegetarian meat substitutes, and legumes
- Low-fat dairy products
- Low- and medium-carb vegetables (see the lists on page 62)
- Salad vegetables
- Fruit (fresh, plain frozen, or canned without added sugar)
- High-carb (starchy) vegetables in appropriate portions (see the list on page 62)
- Whole-grain breads, cereals, and pasta in limited portions
- Healthful high-fat foods like nuts, seeds, and avocadoes in moderation
- Healthful fats like olive oil, canola oil, trans-fatty acid–free margarine, and low-sugar salad dressings in moderation

(See Chapter 5 for more details on acceptable foods.)

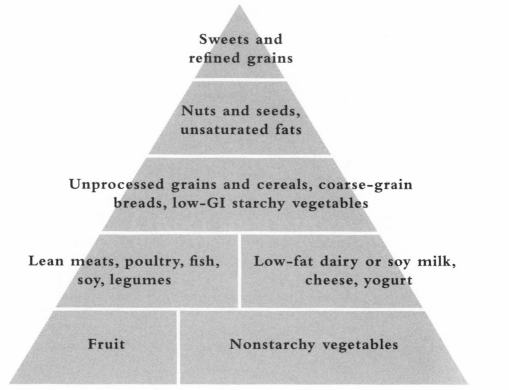

GOOD-CARB LIFE PLAN PRYAMID

Good-Carb Life Plan Menus

WEEK 1	BREAKFAST	LUNCH	SNACK	DINNER
Day 1	1 Sausage & Egg Breakfast Pita (page 133) 1 cup cantaloupe 1 cup nonfat or low-fat milk	Fast food meal: Grilled chicken sandwich on multigrain bun Side salad with 2 Tbsp. light ranch dressing	1 medium apple 1 ounce low-fat cheese	1 serving Savory Stuffed Pork Chops (page 171) ¾ cup Savory Collard Greens (page 213) ½ cup Carrot-Pecan Salad (page 198)
Day 2	1 Peach Passion Smoothie (page 134)	1 Dilly Tuna Salad Sandwich (page 228) Fresh veggies with 2 Tbsp. light ranch dressing	1 cup sugar-free chocolate milk 3 Tbsp. almonds	1 serving Sicilian Stuffed Chicken Breast (page 155) 1 serving Stuffed Portobello Mushrooms (page 215) Garden salad with 1 Tbsp. light olive oil vinaigrette dressing
Day 3	1 Molasses Bran Muffin (page 139) 1 hard-boiled egg 1 cup nonfat or low-fat milk	1 serving Bistro Chicken Salad (page 188)	8 ounces light yogurt	Steak House Restaurant: Grilled steak and veggie kebab 1 small sweet potato with 1 tsp margarine or butter Side salad with 2 Tbsp. light ranch dressing
Day 4	Greek Spinach Omelet (page 124) 1 turkey breakfast sausage patty	1 serving Seafood Cobb Salad (page 190)	1½ oz. low-fat cheese 1 medium apple	1 Burger Dijon (page 231) ¾ cup Green Bean & Tomato Salad (page 199)

	BREAKFAST	LUNCH	SNACK	DINNER
Day 4 *(continued)*	1 cup sliced mango and strawberries			1 serving Cherry Pudding Parfait (page 242)
Day 5	2 slices Light French Toast (page 136), topped with ½ sliced banana, ½ cup blueberries, and 1 Tbsp. honey 2 slices turkey bacon 1 cup nonfat or low-fat milk	Fast food Restaurant: Mandarin grilled chicken salad topped with 2 Tbsp. sliced almonds and 2 Tbsp. Asian dressing (omit the rice noodles)	½ cup nonfat or low-fat cottage cheese 1 peach half canned in juice 1 Tbsp. honey crunch wheat germ	1 serving Lemon Chicken (page 161) 1 cup Spring Vegetable Medley (page 214) 1 serving Roasted Beet Salad with Blue Cheese & Walnuts (page 197)
Day 6	1 serving Microwave Egg Scramble (page 127) 1 cup mixed fresh berries 1 cup nonfat or low-fat milk	1½ cups Beef & Barley Soup (page 143) 1 serving Sunshine Spinach Salad (page 196)	1 piece low-fat string cheese 1 cup grapes 2 Tbsp. walnuts	1 serving Quick Chicken Cacciatore (page 158) with ½ cup whole-wheat spaghetti ¾ cup Broccoli with Garlic & Olive oil (page 211) Garden salad with 1 Tbsp. light Italian dressing
Day 7	1 serving Huevos Rancheros (page 132) 1 cup fresh orange and grapefruit sections 1 cup nonfat or low-fat milk	1½ cups Mediterranean Tuna Pasta Salad (page 202) over fresh salad greens	3 Tbsp. mixed nuts 1½ ounces low-fat cheese	1 serving Cider-Glazed Chicken (page 159) ½ cup Rosemary Roasted Carrots (page 212) ¾ cup Spring Vegetable Pilaf (page 220)

Week 2	Breakfast	Lunch	Snack	Dinner
Day 1	1 cup high-fiber cereal with 1 cup nonfat or low-fat milk and ½ cup fresh blueberries 1 hard-boiled egg	1 Pesto Turkey Wrap (page 232) 1 cup Italian Vegetable Soup (page 149)	1 cup fresh cherries	Seafood Restaurant: 5 ounces grilled or blackened salmon Double order of steamed or grilled veggies Side salad with 1 Tbsp. vinaigrette dressing
Day 2	Restaurant: Western Omelet made with egg substitute Fresh mixed fruit cup 1 cup nonfat or low-fat milk	1 serving Cheesy Crab Melt (page 229) Fresh veggies with 2 Tbsp. light blue cheese dressing	2 celery stalks with ¼ cup hummus	1 serving Mushroom Meatloaf (page 163) ¾ cup Zucchini Pomodoro (page 219) 1 serving Spaghetti Squash with Pesto (page 217) 1 Light Root-Beer Float (page 252)
Day 3	Cantaloupe half filled with ¾ cup low-fat cottage cheese and 1 Tbsp. honey crunch wheat germ	1 cup Cilantro Shrimp Salad (page 194) over mixed baby salad greens 1 cup Savory Butternut Squash Soup (page 150)	½ peanut butter and banana sandwich on whole-grain bread 1 cup nonfat or low-fat milk	Pizza Restaurant: 2 slices thin-crust pizza with vegetable toppings Side salad with 1 Tbsp. Italian dressing
Day 4	Italian Sausage Frittata (page 129) Fresh mixed fruit cup 1 cup nonfat or low-fat milk	1 serving California Chicken Pita (page 227) Fresh raw veggies with 2 Tbsp. light ranch dressing	1 ounce low-fat cheese 1 medium pear	Seared Citrus Scallops (page 176) over a bed of sautéed spinach ¾ cup Cauliflower with Fresh Herbs (page 212) 1 serving Raspberry-Walnut Garden Salad (page 195)

WEEK 2	BREAKFAST	LUNCH	SNACK	DINNER
Day 5	1 poached egg on 1 slice whole-grain toast ½ grapefruit 1 cup nonfat or low-fat milk	1 serving Southwestern Chicken Chop Salad (page 186) 1 cup Zesty Gazpacho (page 148)	8 ounces light yogurt	1 serving Penne with Italian Sausage & Spring Vegetables (page 181) Garden salad with 2 Tbsp. light vinaigrette dressing
Day 6	1 cup cooked oatmeal (½ cup dry) topped with 1 Tbsp. each raisins and walnuts 1 cup nonfat or low-fat milk 1 hard-boiled egg	1 California Club Wrap (page 232) ⅔ cup Colorful Coleslaw (page 195)	Medium apple, sliced and spread with 1 Tbsp. peanut butter	1 serving Broiled Fish with Pesto (page 179) ¾ cup Pilaf with Zucchini & Sun-Dried Tomatoes (page 220) Spinach salad topped with 2 Tbsp. light vinaigrette and 2 Tbsp. low-fat feta cheese
Day 7	1 serving Eggs Sardou (page 132) 2 vegetarian sausage links 1 cup mixed fresh berries	1½ cups Sicilian Vegetable Beef Soup (page 142) 2 celery stalks filled with 1 Tbsp. each light herb cream cheese	8 ounces light yogurt 2 Tbsp. almonds	1 serving Savory Slow-Cooked Brisket (page 169) ¾ cup Herb-Roasted Potatoes, Onions, & Mushrooms (page 218) ¾ cup Caraway Cabbage (page 211) Sliced fresh tomatoes 1 serving Creamy Chocolate Custard (page 243)

General Guidelines for the Good-Carb Life Plan

✦ Include some protein (lean meats, poultry, seafood, dairy, or vegetarian alternatives) in meals.

✦ Fill at least half your plate with vegetables, salads, and fruits at meals.

✦ Choose lower-carb vegetables more often than high-carb ones.

✦ Eat at least three times each day.

✦ Include some protein in snacks.

Calorie Considerations

As with the Low-Carb Quick-Start Plan, foods on the Good-Carb Life Plan are very filling and satisfying, so most people can get excellent results simply by eat-

Low-Carb Loopholes

For many years, going on a low-carb diet meant eating only meat, poultry, fish, fats, and vegetables. Depending on the degree of carbohydrate restriction, some low-carb diets also allowed limited portions of fresh fruit and whole grains. All that has recently changed, though, with a plethora of "low-carb" foods flooding the marketplace.

Now, low-carb dieters are enticed by cookies, brownies, candy, bread, muffins, pasta, and other formerly forbidden foods. These products boast of having only a few "net carbs" per serving. (For more about "net carbs" see the inset on page 82.) But buyer beware: many of these foods contain just as many or even more calories than the foods they are meant to replace! And if you eat more calories than you burn—you *will* store them as fat.

Another thing to think about is that many low-carb products are poor substitutes for the real thing and do little to satisfy a craving. Furthermore, some of these foods cost several times more than the real thing, trimming your wallet instead of your waistline. The moral of this story is that you should always read labels and compare calories. You may be better off eating a small amount of what you really want.

Eat to Lose

If skipping meals is one of your weight-loss strategies you should know that this can backfire in a big way. In fact, a recent study showed that people who eat four times a day are about half as likely to be obese as people who eat less often. Even more remarkable, people who regularly skipped breakfast were 4½ times more likely to be obese.

ing until they are comfortably full without counting calories, carbs, or fat grams. The Good-Carb Life Plan menus on pages 40–43 provide about 1,300 to 1,400 calories per day, and can serve as a good starting point for planning your own personal regimen for weight loss. Keep in mind the guidelines mentioned on page 44: most women should eat at least 1,200 calories per day and most men should eat eat least 1,500 calories. Refer back to Chapter 2 for more about determining your personal calorie needs for weight loss and weight maintenance.

MAKING YOUR DIET WORK FOR YOU

As you work toward changing your diet for the better, it's important to keep in mind that one diet does not fit all. People have very different food preferences, lifestyles, genetics, and physical activity levels. Some trial and error will be necessary to create an eating plan that works for you. For instance, someone who is very physically active will most likely feel better on a diet that is higher in carbohydrate than someone who is sedentary. Chapter 7 explains why and elaborates on the carbohydrate-exercise connection. Some people prefer to eat only three times a day, while others need to eat five or six times a day. And above all, it's important to build your diet around healthful foods that you enjoy eating. Experiment to discover what works best for you.

Taming a Sweet Tooth

Are sweets the downfall of your diet? You *can* learn to tone down a sweet tooth. Soon after starting a healthy lower-carb regimen, most people begin to feel more energized and their craving for sweets begins to lessen. Your blood sugar begins to stabilize, and your taste buds readjust to the more subtle flavors of wholesome natural foods. You will soon develop a new appreciation for the simple sweetness of fruits. After a while, many people begin to find foods like candy and sodas to be sickeningly sweet.

Should you try to never eat sweets again? No. Just save them for special occasions. Also, realize that most of the enjoyment comes from the first few bites. So learn to have just a couple of bites and get most of the pleasure for minimal calories.

Don't believe you can tame your sweet tooth? Ask anyone who has cut back on salt or switched from whole milk to low-fat. After a while, foods like high-sodium canned soup and whole milk taste overpoweringly unpleasant. The same principle applies to sugar. So realize that tastes can change, given the chance. Just hang in there long enough to let it happen.

MOVING TOWARD WEIGHT MAINTENANCE

Any diet plan that cuts your calorie intake will produce weight loss. Keeping the weight off is the real challenge—and this happens only when people make permanent changes in eating and exercise habits.

As you continue to lose weight and then move toward weight maintenance, you can progress your diet by gradually increasing portions and adding occasional treats until you reach a calorie level that sustains your goal weight. This book repeatedly emphasizes that one diet does not fit all, and it's important to find an eating pattern that works for you.

Some people will find that the reduced-carb eating pattern depicted in the

Good-Carb Life Plan pyramid on page 39 is a good fit for keeping their weight in check and maintaining optimal control over blood cholesterol, triglycerides, and glucose. This pattern emphasizes nonstarchy vegetables, fruits, and lean proteins as mainstays of the diet. Starchy vegetables, breads, and cereals are also allowed, in limited portions.

Others will find that they can enjoy a higher proportion of carbohydrate in their maintenance diet—as long as they remain physically active and choose predominately low-GI good carbs. The following pyramid illustrates a more liberalized approach to the Good-Carb Life Plan, still emphasizing nonstarchy vegetables, fruits, and lean proteins, but allowing for more moderate portions of starchy vegetables and grain products. For a personalized nutrition prescription, you can consult with a registered dietitian who specializes in weight management.

Sweets and
junk food

Nuts and seeds,
unsaturated fats

Lean meats, poultry, fish,
eggs, soy, legumes

Low-fat dairy or soy milk,
cheese, yogurt

Unprocessed grains and cereals,
coarse-grain breads, starchy vegetables

Fruit

Nonstarchy vegetables

LIBERALIZED GOOD-CARB LIFE PLAN PRYAMID

CURBING CARBOHYDRATE CRAVINGS AND BINGES

Cravings almost always center on high-carb, high-fat foods. Women tend to crave chocolate, ice cream, cookies, and other sweets, while men usually long for foods like chips, French fries, and pizza. What causes food cravings? It's commonly believed that we instinctively crave foods that supply needed nutrients. A yearning for chocolate, for instance, might indicate that the body needs magnesium. The problem is, if we craved what our bodies really needed, we would be much more likely to binge on a big plate of vegetables!

A more likely explanation is that highly palatable foods cause the brain to release beta-endorphins, the body's natural "feel-good" chemicals. Starches and sugars also raise levels of serotonin, a neurotransmitter that has a calming effect. See the inset "Can You Be Addicted to Carbohydrate?" on page 27 for more information.

What's the best way to keep cravings under control? Addressing the root of the problem offers the only real hope for a permanent solution. Here are some tips.

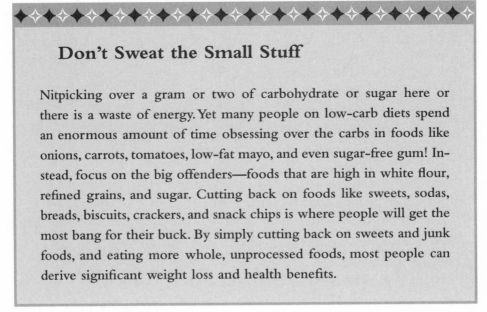

Don't Sweat the Small Stuff

Nitpicking over a gram or two of carbohydrate or sugar here or there is a waste of energy. Yet many people on low-carb diets spend an enormous amount of time obsessing over the carbs in foods like onions, carrots, tomatoes, low-fat mayo, and even sugar-free gum! Instead, focus on the big offenders—foods that are high in white flour, refined grains, and sugar. Cutting back on foods like sweets, sodas, breads, biscuits, crackers, and snack chips is where people will get the most bang for their buck. By simply cutting back on sweets and junk foods, and eating more whole, unprocessed foods, most people can derive significant weight loss and health benefits.

Prioritize Your Eating Plan

Understanding the role that high-GI carbs play in triggering hunger is fundamental for curbing cravings and binge eating. Eating well-spaced meals and snacks that include protein and fiber-rich foods will maintain more stable blood sugar levels and help keep you feeling full and satisfied. This means you will be less likely to eat when you're not hungry.

De-stress

It's no secret that stress is a major cause of overeating. And it's not tuna fish and salad that stressed-out people crave—it's cookies, ice cream, and chips. Why does stress send many people seeking sugary, fatty foods? When stress strikes, the body releases various hormones that enable it to cope. One of these hormones, *cortisol,* triggers appetite and favors fat storage around the belly.

As discussed in Chapter 3, stressed-out people also get some relief from eating carbs, which raise serotonin and endorphin levels and produce a feeling of well-being. You can see why finding ways to simplify your life, learning to relax, and dealing with emotional issues are just as important as nutrition and exercise when it comes to weight-loss success. So the next time stress strikes, bear in mind that "STRESSED" spelled backwards is "DESSERTS"!

Don't Obsess

Putting any particular food off limits can make you crave it even more and lead to unhealthy food obsessions and bingeing. This is because obsessing about diet and weight loss can stress you out—leading to all of the stress-related reactions described above that make weight loss nearly impossible. You will be much better off if you can maintain a relaxed attitude, focus on eating well for good health, be patient, and be content with gradual but steady weight loss.

Enjoy an Occasional Splurge

Most people find that they can still enjoy the foods they crave if they include them in a controlled manner. For instance, go out for ice cream every now and then instead of keeping it in your home freezer where you will be more likely to overindulge. If you keep treats at home, store them out of sight. Portion them out and put the package away before you begin to eat. Never eat the food right out of the package. When you do have a treat, really take the time to enjoy and savor it. Then get right back on your program.

Case Study: Plateau Problems

After seven weeks on a lower-carb eating plan, Joyce had lost 18 pounds. However, her weight loss had recently stalled, and had started creeping back up over the past several weeks. Becoming very discouraged, Joyce consulted with a registered dietitian to see what she could do. She began writing down everything she ate and drank, and was amazed at what she discovered.

Her typical breakfast consisted of two eggs cooked in olive oil with some full-fat cheese and two slices of bacon. Mid-morning snack was two stalks of celery filled with peanut butter or a couple of ounces of cheese. Lunch was usually a large salad topped with grilled chicken and a generous amount of vinaigrette dressing. This was followed by an afternoon snack of ½ cup of mixed nuts. Dinner typically consisted of 6 ounces of meat, sautéed vegetables, and a salad with blue-cheese dressing.

Lately, Joyce had started to "crave carbohydrates," was having problems with low energy, and generally felt like she was "missing something." She started eating some sugar-free candies and chocolate bars, and nibbling on other high-carb sweets that her husband kept in the house.

By keeping a record of her food intake, Joyce discovered that she was eating close to 2,500 calories on most days—about 500 calories more than she needed to sustain her current weight of 145 pounds. She found that nuts and salad dressing alone were adding nearly 800 calories to her daily diet! In addition, she discovered that her sugar-free treats contained just as many calories as the "real thing."

Joyce's dietitian helped her revamp her diet. She switched to reduced-fat cheeses, cut back to more moderate amounts of peanut butter, nuts, and salad dressing. She found ways to work some "good carbs" into her diet, such as a sandwich in whole-wheat pita bread at lunch, some fruit with breakfast, and light yogurt for a snack. She was even allowed an occasional treat of a small piece of "real" chocolate or a few chocolate-covered almonds. These changes brought her calorie intake down to about 1,500 per day, while still keeping her carb intake moderately low.

Almost immediately, Joyce began to feel better and her cravings subsided. She felt like she was eating more food than before, and she was much more satisfied. Her weight started coming down at the rate of about one pound per week. Her energy level increased, and she was able to step up her exercise routine a bit. Her newly modified plan was much better suited for long-term success.

Find Lower-Calorie Substitutions

Treats like sugar-free hot cocoa, a light fudge pop, or a root-beer float made with light ice cream and sugar-free soda can help satisfy a sweet tooth for only a few calories.

Get Plenty of Rest

For many people, the key to better weight control might just lie in a good night's sleep. Why? People who feel fatigued during the day often snack in an effort to gain energy and increase alertness. Lack of sleep also increases the body's production of cortisol, the stress hormone discussed above, which triggers hunger. This is why people who are sleep deprived often feel hungry despite getting enough to eat.

Altered hormone levels that result from sleep deprivation can also impair carbohydrate metabolism, leading to higher blood sugar and insulin levels and increased fat storage. As if that's not bad enough, lack of sleep is also associated with lower levels of growth hormone, so people who are sleep deprived may have a harder time building and maintaining lean body mass.

The bottom line is sleep deprivation can put on pounds. You can eat well and exercise with the best of intentions, but if you don't get enough rest, you won't get the maximum benefit from your weight-loss attempts.

Spend Time Outdoors

Being deprived of natural sunlight can alter the body's levels of serotonin and melatonin. This causes some people to feel lethargic and depressed, and to crave carbohydrates. These feelings become even more of a problem in the winter months when the days are shorter and can lead to a condition known as seasonal affective disorder (SAD). So make an effort to get outside during your breaks at work, go for a walk when you get off work, and plan outdoor activities like gardening, biking, and hiking on the weekend. These simple strategies can provide a powerful boost to your weight-management and total-wellness program.

SECRETS OF LONG-TERM SUCCESS

A healthy lower-carb eating plan can get you on the road to weight-loss success. But how do you keep it off long-term? Researchers are currently studying a group of people who have done just that. The National Weight Control Registry is evaluating the habits of successful losers to see what habits are responsible for their success. The average NWCR participant has lost over 60 pounds and kept it off for six years. How do they do it? So far, researchers have identified the following habits of successful "losers."

Eat Breakfast

People who are trying to lose weight often skip breakfast, thinking this is a good way to cut calories. This is a bad idea. For one thing, eating breakfast revs up your metabolism so you burn more calories earlier in the day. For another, skipping breakfast just sets you up to feel hungry and overeat later in the day.

Many people also skip breakfast because it makes them feel hungry all day long. If this sounds familiar, you're probably eating the wrong breakfast. Breakfast foods like cereal bars, toaster pastries, bagels, and many cereals are loaded with refined carbs. These foods can wreak havoc on your blood sugar, trigger hunger, and set the tone for overeating all day long. But rather than skip breakfast, choose a better breakfast—featuring fiber-rich foods and lean proteins. Chapters 5 and 9 present plenty of ideas that will keep you feeling full and satisfied all morning long.

Watch Fat Intake

Successful losers lose their weight by a variety of means, but most maintain their weight loss with a sensible diet. The average NWCR participant eats a modest 25 percent of their calories as fat. They avoid fried foods, choose lean meats and low-fat dairy products, and replace other fatty foods with lighter versions. About half of their calories come from carbohydrate and about 20 percent from protein. This should provide some reassurance that as you reach your weight-loss goal, it's okay to liberalize your carb intake a little—as long as you stick with mostly unrefined "good" carbs and as long as your levels of cholesterol, triglycerides, and blood sugar remain within the desirable range.

Exercise for an Hour a Day

Successful weight-loss maintainers burn about 2,700 calories a week in physical activity, the equivalent of about a four-mile walk daily. Regular exercise improves insulin sensitivity, which lowers blood insulin levels and improves blood glucose and cholesterol levels. This is why active people can consume higher levels of dietary carbohydrate than their sedentary counterparts without experiencing the adverse effects.

Monitor Weight Frequently and Keep Track of Food Intake

Ignorance is not bliss. Monitoring your weight, either by weighing yourself periodically or by being aware of how your clothes fit, allows you to catch problems early and do something about them. Keeping track of what and how much you eat keeps you focused and helps prevent "portion distortion" and "carb creep."

❖❖❖❖❖

Do successful losers find weight maintenance a chore? Most find that the longer they keep their weight off the easier it becomes, as their new habits become more firmly ingrained.

5.

Stocking the Carb-Conscious Pantry

Never before has it been so easy to eat well on a carbohydrate-controlled diet. With interest in low-carb diets at an all-time high, a barrage of new products is available to choose from. Unfortunately, things are not always what they seem, and trouble may loom ahead for the unwary consumer. In the pages that follow, we'll take a look at the lean meats, low-fat dairy products, eggs and egg substitutes, spreads and dressings, produce items, and many other foods that will ensure success in all your carb-conscious cooking and eating adventures.

MEAT, POULTRY, AND SEAFOOD

Including some protein in meals and snacks is key to success on your lower-carb eating plan. For one thing, these foods are carbohydrate-free—unless they are sugar-cured, soaked in a sweet marinade, or glazed with a sweet sauce. For another, protein-rich foods help stabilize your blood sugar and delay the return of hunger between meals. In addition, eating adequate protein will help you preserve muscle and maintain a higher metabolic rate as you lose weight.

Protein—How Much Is Enough?

The *minimum* recommended amount of protein for healthy adults is about 0.4 grams per pound of ideal body weight, or about 60 grams for a 150-pound person. There is growing evidence that people over age fifty may need as much as 0.5 to 0.6 grams per pound. Athletes also need extra protein. Low-carb diets typically provide 1½ to 2 times the minimum recommended amount, which covers the needs of virtually anyone.

While it's important to include some protein with meals and snacks, there's no need to go overboard. A general guideline is to include a serving of protein the size of your palm (3 to 5 ounces) in meals, and have a serving size equal to one or two fingers (an ounce or two) with snacks. You can get your protein from a variety of foods, including lean meats, skinless poultry, seafood, low-fat cheese and milk, legumes, tofu, and vegetarian meat alternatives.

Protein Content of Selected Foods

Food	Amount	Protein (grams)
Chicken, fish, beef, pork	3 ounces cooked	21
Legumes	1 cup cooked	14
Tofu	3 ounces	13
Vegetarian burger	2½ ounces	6–12
Vegetarian breakfast sausage	1½ ounces	8–10
Milk	1 cup	8
Cheese	1 ounce	8
Bread (regular)	1 slice	2–3
Bread (low-carb)	1 slice	4–8
Rice, pasta, grains	½ cup cooked	3
Vegetables	½ cup cooked	2
Fruit	1 piece	<1

Fish—Health Food or Health Hazard?

High in protein and beneficial omega-3 fatty acids, fish has long been considered one of the ultimate health foods. Fish consumption has been associated with a reduced risk of many health problems, including heart disease, dementia, and Alzheimer's. Unfortunately, reports of contamination from mercury and polychlorinated biphenyls (PCBs) have cast a shadow over fish consumption. Exposure to excess mercury can cause nerve damage, and PCBs have been linked to cancer. These pollutants enter waters from coal and waste incineration, pulp and paper manufacturing, and other industrial processes.

Toxins accumulate as they pass up the food chain, so longer-lived predatory fish such as shark, swordfish, tilefish, and king mackerel contain the highest amounts and pose the biggest health threat. Recently, tuna steaks and canned albacore tuna have been added to the list of fish that may contain unhealthy amounts of mercury. (Light tuna typically contains less mercury because it is a smaller fish.) And concerns have also been raised about farmed salmon, which may contain much higher levels of pollutants than wild salmon.

What's the bottom line? The benefits of eating fish still outweigh the risks. To limit your exposure to harmful substances, avoid the previously mentioned large predatory fish and eat a variety of different fishes instead of having the same kind over and over. PCBs are especially concentrated in the fatty portions, so trimming away the skin and fat will reduce your exposure—of course, this also eliminates some of the omega-3 fatty acids. Mercury is distributed all throughout the fish, so removing the skin and fat will not diminish the mercury content. You can get updates on the latest recommendations by visiting the FDA (www.fda.gov) and EPA (www.epa.gov) websites.

Should You Supplement?

People who don't eat fish might consider a fish-oil supplement. A supplement of up to 1 gram of omega-3 fatty acids per day is generally considered safe with minimal risk for side effects. Depending on the product, up to three fish-oil capsules will provide 1 gram per day of the omega-3 fats EPA and DHA. It's important to read labels to make sure you are getting the right dose.

A word of warning: Taking fish oil may be contraindicated if you are taking certain medications. And doses higher than 1 gram of omega-3 fatty acids per day could present problems with prolonged bleeding, higher LDL ("bad") cholesterol levels, elevated blood glucose, and gastrointestinal upset, so should be taken only with your physician's guidance.

Of course, not all high-protein foods are alike, so be sure to choose the lean foods listed below to keep calories and saturated fat at a minimum. Bear in mind that processed meats like ham, luncheon meats, and hot dogs are high in sodium, so eat these foods less often. Be sure to eat fish at least twice a week, and frequently substitute vegetarian alternatives for meat.

✦   Skinless chicken and turkey
✦   Rotisserie chicken (remove the skin)
✦   Precooked grilled chicken breasts and strips
✦   "Heat and eat" ready-made entrées like pot roast, turkey and gravy, or brisket (Look for items with no more than 3 to 5 grams of fat per serving.)
✦   Frozen entrées made with lean meat or poultry and vegetables.
✦   Marinated ready-to-cook pork and turkey tenderloins (Avoid those packed in sweet marinades.)
✦   Ready-to-cook kabobs made with chicken or lean beef
✦   Ground turkey (Look for ground turkey that is at least 95 percent lean.)
✦   Beef round or sirloin, London broil, flat half brisket
✦   Ground beef (Look for ground beef that is 93 to 96 percent lean.)
✦   Pork tenderloin, loin roast, or chops
✦   Ham (Look for ham that is at least 95 percent lean.)
✦   Turkey bacon (Tip: For a crisp texture, cook turkey bacon in a microwave oven; for a chewy texture, cook in a skillet.)

✦ Canadian bacon
✦ Smoked sausage and kielbasa (Look for products that are at least 95 to 97 percent lean.)
✦ Luncheon meats and hot dogs (Look for products that are at least 95 to 97 percent lean.)
✦ Assorted fresh fish and shellfish (See the inset on page 56 for more on choosing fish and seafood.)
✦ Canned tuna, salmon, and crab packed in spring water or pouches
✦ Sardines packed in mustard or tomato sauce
✦ Precooked (steamed) shrimp
✦ Frozen cooked shrimp

VEGETARIAN MEAT ALTERNATIVES

Adopting a lower-carb diet does not necessarily mean eating large quantities of meat—there are plenty of meatless alternatives available to choose from. And even if you are a sworn meat eater, you should include more plant sources of protein in your repertoire. These products are cholesterol-free, low in saturated fat, and provide a variety of nutrients that animal products do not. In addition, since plant foods are lower on the food chain, they typically contain fewer environmental contaminants, like dioxins and agricultural chemicals, which bioaccumulate up the food chain—and are especially concentrated in the fatty portions of meat and dairy products. And, of course, growing plant foods consumes and pollutes far fewer natural resources than does raising animals for food.

Most vegetarian meat alternatives are quite low in carbs. The exception is legumes. However, legumes are exceptionally high in fiber, and their carbohydrate is slowly absorbed, giving them a very low glycemic index.

✦ Veggie burgers
✦ Vegetarian hamburger crumbles and texturized vegetable protein (TVP)
✦ Veggie breakfast sausage and bacon
✦ Tofu
✦ Legumes, such as dried or canned black, pinto, navy, white, and garbanzo beans; dried or canned black-eyed peas, dried or canned split peas and lentils; and green soybeans (edamame)

DAIRY PRODUCTS

Many low-carb diet plans strictly prohibit milk because it contains carbohydrate (about 12 grams per cup). Instead they recommend pure cream, which is very low in carbohydrate. Carbohydrate content aside, cream has eight times the calories of nonfat milk and is loaded with artery-clogging saturated fat.

If you like milk, *do* include it in your diet. The sugar in milk (lactose) has a very low glycemic index, so it has a minimal impact on blood sugar levels. In addition, milk and other dairy foods like yogurt and cheese are an excellent source of high-quality protein, which helps prevent between-meal hunger. Recent studies have also found that people who consume two to three servings of dairy products daily have less body fat, have lower blood pressure, and are less likely to be insulin resistant.

Need another reason to choose low-fat dairy products? Environmental toxins such as dioxins and pesticides concentrate in the fatty portions of meats and dairy products, so choosing lower-fat versions can reduce your exposure to these harmful substances.

- ✦ Nonfat or low-fat milk
- ✦ Nonfat or low-fat buttermilk
- ✦ Evaporated nonfat or low-fat milk
- ✦ Calcium-fortified soy milk
- ✦ Light (no added sugar) yogurt
- ✦ Nonfat or low-fat cottage cheese
- ✦ Nonfat or reduced-fat ricotta cheese
- ✦ Reduced-fat cheddar, Colby, mozzarella, Monterey Jack, provolone, Swiss, etc.
- ✦ Parmesan and blue cheese (These cheeses are high in fat but since a little goes a long way, they can be enjoyed in moderation.)
- ✦ Reduced-fat feta cheese

Calcium and Body Weight

Because many low-carb diets discourage foods like milk and yogurt, they are often woefully deficient in calcium. Unfortunately, this nit-picking over carbs may actually work against your weight-loss efforts. How? Mounting evidence suggests that high-calcium diets fight obesity by encouraging the body to burn fat rather than store it.

One study found that each 300-milligram increase in daily calcium intake (the equivalent of one cup of milk) was associated with about 2 pounds less body fat in children and 5 to 6 pounds less body fat in adults. Another study found that people who included yogurt in their daily diet lost more weight in the stomach area and were about twice as effective at maintaining muscle mass as people who consumed low-dairy, low-calcium diets. Besides speeding weight loss, low-fat dairy foods have been shown to help reduce high blood pressure and may protect against insulin resistance. And of course, a high-calcium diet helps to maintain strong bones.

What's the best way to get your calcium? The fat-fighting and health benefits of calcium appear to be greatest when consumed in foods rather than in supplements. Dairy products such as low-fat milk, yogurt, and cheese are an excellent source—aim for two to three servings per day. Other calcium-rich foods include greens, calcium-fortified soy foods, and legumes. If necessary, take enough supplemental calcium to bring your intake up to the recommended daily amount. Adults up to age fifty should aim for 1,000 milligrams per day. After age fifty, the calcium requirement increases to 1,200 milligrams per day.

EGGS

Quick and easy to prepare, eggs are a natural for lower-carb diets. And egg yolks are rich in lutein and zeaxanthin, two carotenoids that may help prevent macular degeneration. But because eggs are also high in cholesterol, whether or not they should be included in a heart-healthy diet has been a long-standing controversy.

What should you do? The preponderance of evidence indicates that an egg a day does not significantly raise blood cholesterol or the risk of heart disease for most people. Furthermore, cutting back on saturated and trans fats is much more effective at lowering blood cholesterol than is avoiding high-cholesterol foods like eggs. That said, some people are sensitive to dietary cholesterol and may need to limit cholesterol-rich foods like egg yolks. Consult with your physician or dietitian for more specific advice.

When you do choose whole eggs, look for omega-3-enriched brands. These eggs come from chickens that eat a diet enriched with ingredients like flax and marine algae, which raises the omega-3 content of their egg yolks. Egg whites and fat-free egg substitutes can be eaten freely, since they contain no fat or cholesterol at all.

- ✦ Omega-3-enriched eggs
- ✦ Egg whites
- ✦ Fat-free egg substitutes

VEGETABLES

Loaded with fiber and disease-fighting nutrients, vegetables should be a central part of your carb-conscious eating plan. With a few exceptions, most vegetables are quite low in carbohydrate and calories. Be sure to eat a wide variety of different colors of vegetables (and fruits) because different pigments—green, yellow/orange, red, blue/purple, and white—indicate the presence of different types of phytochemicals that fight cancer, heart disease, and numerous other health problems.

Unfortunately, many low-carb diet plans needlessly restrict consumption of vegetables. For instance, you may see advice to avoid foods like carrots, beets, rutabaga, onions, tomatoes, and even zucchini, red bell peppers, and broccoli. This is not only silly; it can compromise your health. No one ever got fat from eating vegetables. In fact, studies show that people who eat generous portions of a wide variety of vegetables are thinner than people who restrict these foods.

The exception is for high-carb (starchy) vegetables such as potatoes, corn, baked beans, lima beans, and peas, which are higher in calories. Think of starchy vegetables as bread or rice substitutes and include them in your diet as your carbohydrate and calorie budgets allow. Below you will find a breakdown of vegetables according to their carbohydrate content.

Seven to ten servings of vegetables and fruits every day will provide a generous amount of health-promoting nutrients. If you are following the Low-Carb Quick-Start Plan, you will rely mainly on low-carb vegetables for these nutrients. The Good-Carb Life Plan will expand your selection of produce to also include fruit.

Very-Low-Carb Vegetables
(<5 grams of carbohydrate per serving):
Fresh spinach, lettuce, arugula, and other salad greens; raw salad vegetables such as broccoli (1 cup), cauliflower, celery, cucumbers, mushrooms, peppers, radishes, scallions, and sprouts.

Low-Carb (Nonstarchy) Vegetables
(approximately 5 grams of carbohydrate per serving):
Artichokes, asparagus, bamboo shoots, bean sprouts, broccoli (½ cup), broccoli rabe (rapini), green beans, Brussels sprouts, cabbage, carrots, cauliflower, eggplant, green beans, collard and mustard greens, hearts of palm, jicama, kale, kohlrabi, leeks, okra, snow peas, bell peppers, pumpkin, spinach, spaghetti squash, yellow squash, tomatillos, tomatoes, turnips and turnip greens, and zucchini.

Medium-Carb Vegetables
(approximately 10 grams of carbohydrate per serving):
Beets, onions, rutabaga, sugar snap peas, and water chestnuts.

High-Carb (Starchy) Vegetables
(approximately 15 grams of carbohydrate per serving):
Corn, baked beans, lima beans, black-eyed peas, legumes, green peas, small new potatoes, sweet potatoes, baking potatoes, acorn squash, butternut squash,

and yams. (Within this group, baked and mashed potatoes have the highest GI, and baked beans usually contain added sugar, so choose these less often.)

Now that you understand where specific vegetables rank on the carbohydrate continuum, it's time to load up your shopping cart. Here are some vegetable and produce items to look for.

✦ Assorted fresh salad greens and salad vegetables
✦ Assorted fresh and plain frozen low-carb vegetables
✦ Medium- and high-carb vegetables as your eating plan allows

Vegetables and Fruits—What's a Serving?

Five servings of fruits and vegetables a day is the recommended minimum. But to optimize your health, aim for seven to ten servings every day. This is not as hard as you may think, since each of the following constitutes a serving:

✦ 1 cup leafy salad greens
✦ ½ cup cooked or raw fruit or vegetables
✦ ½ cup cooked dried beans or peas
✦ 1 medium piece of fruit such as an apple, peach, or orange
✦ ¼ cup dried fruit
✦ ¾ cup fruit or vegetable juice

Using the above guidelines, a large chef salad made with 3 cups of lettuce plus a cup of other chopped vegetables like mushrooms, onions, carrots, and tomatoes equals five servings. A meal that contains a cup of steamed broccoli plus a medium baked sweet potato equals four servings. If you include at least one cup of vegetables or fruit at each meal, and replace snacks like pretzels, crackers, chips, and cookies with fruits and vegetables, you will easily meet or exceed the daily recommendation.

✦   Canned vegetables (drain to remove about 40 percent of the sodium)

✦   Assorted prewashed salad greens

✦   Prewashed greens such as collard, turnip, and mustard greens, spinach, and kale

✦   Baby carrots and fresh matchstick carrots

✦   Preshredded coleslaw mix

✦   Broccoli slaw

✦   Cherry and grape tomatoes

✦   Ready-cut vegetables for snacking

✦   Ready-to-cook fresh stir-fry vegetables

✦   Avocadoes (use moderately if you are watching your weight)

FRUITS

The thought of giving up fruit is enough to discourage most people from sticking with a low-carb diet for any length of time. The good news is that there is no need to even consider this as a lifelong weight-control strategy. You will get far more bang for your buck by targeting processed carbs like sweets and sugary sodas. And as you trim the sugar-laden foods from your diet, your taste threshold for sugar will decline. You may be surprised at how much more flavorful and enjoyable fruit becomes.

If you opt for the Low-Carb Quick-Start Plan outlined in Chapter 4, you will give up fruit for a short period of time. However, people who prefer a less stringent approach can certainly add a serving or two of fruit per day and still get good results. The Good-Carb Life Plan in Chapter 4 encourages you to satisfy a sweet tooth with fruit instead of cookies, candy, desserts, and sodas. Just doing this can dramatically reduce your carbohydrate intake. For instance, a medium apple contains about 20 grams of carbohydrate, but a serving of apple pie contains nearly 60 grams.

Are there certain fruits you should avoid? Not really. Fruits like bananas, pineapple, watermelon, and raisins have a higher glycemic load than fruits like apples, peaches, plums, and cherries. But eaten in moderation, even high-GI fruits are healthful choices. When possible, always choose the whole fruit over juice, since liquid calories go down too easy and are not nearly as filling as eating the fiber-rich fruit.

- ✦ Assorted fresh fruits
- ✦ Unsweetened frozen fruit
- ✦ Canned fruit in natural juice
- ✦ Unsweetened applesauce
- ✦ Dried fruits (in moderation)

NUTS AND SEEDS

Though frequently shunned by low-fat dieters, nuts and seeds are embraced by the low-carb crowd—owing to their low glycemic load. The caveat is that nuts are loaded with calories (close to 200 calories per quarter-cup!) and overindulging has proven to be a stumbling block for many people following a low-carb eating plan.

The good news is that, in moderation, nuts can be part of a healthy low-carb diet. In fact, people who eat an ounce of nuts (3 to 4 tablespoons) on most

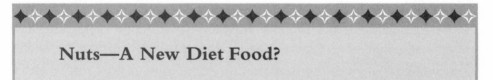

Nuts—A New Diet Food?

It wasn't too long ago that nuts were a big "no-no" for weight-loss diets. Now researchers are taking a new look at how nuts can actually help people lose weight. New studies show that even though nuts are high in fat and calories, they can help people lose weight *and* keep it off. How can this be? High in protein, "good" fats, and fiber, nuts provide a feeling of fullness. On the other hand, high-carb, low-fat "diet foods" like rice cakes, pretzels, and graham crackers can actually stimulate hunger.

Of course, a quarter cup of nuts contains nearly 200 calories, so it's important to *substitute* nuts for other foods such as snack chips and sweets. You can't just add nuts to your daily diet and expect to lose weight. When possible, purchase nuts and seeds in their shells. Having to crack them will slow down the rate at which you eat.

days of the week are a lot less likely to develop heart disease. New studies indicate that nuts may also protect against diabetes. How do nuts confer these health benefits? They are rich in antioxidants and phytochemicals, as well as nutrients like magnesium, copper, folate, and zinc, each of which thwarts a number of health problems.

So if you like nuts, feel free to have a small handful for a snack. Sprinkle a tablespoon or two of walnuts or sliced almonds over salad instead of croutons. Use coarsely chopped or ground nuts as a coating for fish or chicken, or sprinkle some toasted chopped nuts on green beans and other vegetables.

✦   Almonds, cashews, pecans, pine nuts, pistachios, walnuts
✦   Natural peanut butter and other nut butters
✦   Sunflower, pumpkin, and sesame seeds

BREADS, CEREALS, AND GRAIN PRODUCTS

No food group is currently more controversial than this one. Long thought of as "the staff of life," bread, rice, cereal, and pasta form the base of the USDA Food Guide Pyramid, with six to eleven servings recommended daily. However, growing numbers of nutrition experts question whether this food group should play such a large role in our diet. Some even question whether this food group is essential at all.

What's the truth? Grains were virtually absent from the human diet until the appearance of agriculture some 10,000 years ago. Since then, grains have become the primary source of calories for people all over the world. Some believe that we are not genetically adapted to eating such a large proportion of grains. And the consequence of substituting grain products for super-nutritious, lower-calorie foods like vegetables and fruits may be an increased susceptibility to cancer, cardiovascular disease, and other health problems. Allergies and intolerances to wheat and other grains is also an increasingly recognized problem. For instance, an estimated 1 in 250 Americans has a condition known as *celiac disease* or *gluten intolerance*. Celiac is linked to a number of health problems, including type 1 diabetes, osteoporosis, arthritis, and intestinal cancer.

On the other hand, numerous civilizations have thrived on a grain-based diet for thousands of years. For instance, rice has long been a staple in Asian

What About "Low-Carb" Bread and Pasta?

Do you need special foods like low-carb/high-protein bread and pasta to enjoy weight-loss success? Eyeing a growing market, manufacturers are marketing these, plus chips, crackers, and many other foods, that were formerly forbidden on a low-carb eating plan. Here are the facts about these "substitute" foods.

Reduced-carb bread, with about half the carbs of regular bread, has been around for years as "light" bread. But these days, new versions of ultra-low-carb, high-protein bread are also available. Low-carb breads may be made from either white or whole-grain flours combined with soy or wheat protein. They may also contain ingredients like nondigestible starches and fibers, which function as low-glycemic bulking agents. The calories in low-carb bread may or may not be lower than a same-size piece of regular whole-wheat bread.

Low-carb pasta is often made from ingredients like soy, wheat gluten (protein), plant fibers, and eggs, combined with wheat flour, rice flour, or other grains. As with low-carb bread, it may or may not have fewer calories than regular pasta.

What's the bottom line? As usual, it's buyer beware. Regular whole-wheat pasta and dense, whole-grain breads are high in fiber and nutrients and have a low to moderate glycemic index—so there's really no need to look for extreme alternatives. However, if you enjoy the substitute products and don't mind paying a premium price for them, then include them in your diet as your calorie budget allows. But realize that if these products save you few or no calories, they will do nothing to further your weight-loss goals.

countries—whose people enjoy great health and longevity. And pasta has long been a central part of the heart-healthy Mediterranean diet.

What's the take-home message? If you have a weight problem or are insulin resistant, the bulk of your carbohydrate intake should come from foods with a lower glycemic load, like vegetables and fruits. Moderate amounts of minimally processed whole grains and whole-grain breads, cereals, and pasta can also be included in a healthful eating plan, but unless you are very active, six to eleven servings per day is far too much carbohydrate for most people. And, of course, people who have grain allergies or intolerances should first and foremost avoid the offending foods.

People who opt for the Low-Carb Quick-Start Plan will forgo grain products for a short period of time. However, once you progress to the Good-Carb Life Plan, you will be able to add back the following types of grain products.

✦ Whole grains, such as barley, brown rice, bulgur wheat, whole-wheat couscous, kamut, quinoa, spelt, and wild rice
✦ Whole-grain cereals such as old-fashioned oatmeal, oat bran, shredded wheat, bran cereals, and other high-fiber low-sugar cereals; look for at least 5 grams of fiber per 2-ounce serving

Whole Grains—Finding the "Real Thing"

Whole-grain foods are far superior to refined versions. Unfortunately, identifying the "real thing" can be tricky. Why? Products like "natural grain bread" and "golden wheat crackers" may contain far more refined white flour than whole grains. And having a dark brown color does not make a bread whole grain. Here are some clues that can help you hone in on the real thing:

✦ Whole wheat, or another whole grain such as whole rye, or oats should be listed as the *first* ingredient.
✦ Avoid products that list "wheat" or "enriched wheat" as the first ingredient, as these are other names for refined wheat.
✦ Check out the ingredient list, and look for other fiber-rich ingredients like wheat bran, oat bran, oatmeal, wheat berries, cracked wheat, wheat germ, sprouted grains, and flax.
✦ Whole-grain products will have at least 2 grams of fiber per slice of bread, ounce of crackers, or ounce of cereal.

- Hearty 100 percent whole-grain breads, bagels, and burger buns that include ingredients like stone-ground whole-wheat flour, oats, oat bran, wheat berries, cracked wheat, whole rye, sprouted grains, and flaxseeds; look for at least 2 grams of fiber per 1-ounce serving
- Rye and pumpernickel breads—but most brands contain more white flour than whole grain; be sure to check the ingredient list for whole-grain flours and look for at least 2 grams of fiber per slice.
- Lower-carb, high-fiber breads; a wide array of reduced-carb and "light" sandwich breads, burger buns, and hot dog buns are available with about half the carbs of regular bread; look for brands made with whole-grain flours, with at least 2 grams of fiber per 1-ounce serving
- Whole-wheat pasta
- Whole-wheat tortillas
- Corn tortillas; choose thin corn tortillas, which have 25 to 35 calories and 6 to 8 grams of carbohydrate per tortilla, instead of thick tortillas, which have up to twice this amount.
- Chapati (a whole-wheat Indian flatbread similar to a tortilla)
- Whole-grain pita bread
- Whole-grain English muffins
- 100% whole-grain crackers like Finn Crisp, Kavli, Wasa, and reduced-fat Triscuits
- Air-popped or light microwave popcorn (popcorn is a whole grain)

CANNED AND JARRED FOODS

A variety of convenient canned and bottled foods can have a place in both the Low-Carb Quick-Start Plan and the Good-Carb Life Plan. Here are some examples:

- Artichoke—hearts and bottoms, or marinated hearts
- Pickles—dill and sugar-free sweet (in moderation—they are high in sodium)
- Beans such as black, kidney, pinto, navy, garbanzo, black-eyed peas, and chili beans (draining and rinsing removes about 40 percent of the sodium)
- Hearts of palm
- Olives

✦ Peanut butter and nut butters (high in calories, so use in moderation)
✦ Peppers—roasted red bell, hot
✦ Sauerkraut (in moderation—it is high in sodium)
✦ Soups—chicken, turkey, or beef with vegetables; vegetarian vegetable; bean; lentil; split pea; tomato; and low-fat cream soups (choose reduced-sodium brands)
✦ Spaghetti and marinara sauce (look for brands with no added sugar)
✦ Sun-dried tomatoes, plain or packed in olive oil (drain before using)
✦ Tomatoes, stewed tomatoes, tomato sauce, tomato paste
✦ Tomato juice
✦ Tuna, salmon, crab, sardines, anchovies
✦ Vegetable juice cocktail

MAYONNAISE AND SALAD DRESSINGS

Low-carb diet plans often advise people to use only full-fat mayonnaise and salad dressings because lower-fat versions contain sugar or other carbohydrates. While this may be true, the amount of carb in the lower-fat products is usually not enough to worry about, and the calorie savings are considerable. For instance, a tablespoon of nonfat mayonnaise that contains 10 calories and 2 grams of carb is definitely a better choice than a tablespoon of full-fat mayo with 100 calories and 11 grams of fat!

As for salad dressings, some lower-fat brands are loaded with carbs while others are practically carbohydrate-free. Read labels and compare brands for calorie, carb, and fat content. A salad dressing with 3 to 4 grams of carb per 2-tablespoon serving is not unreasonable.

What if you don't like the reduced-fat products? Go ahead and use a full-fat product, just be sure to use it sparingly.

✦ Nonfat and reduced-fat mayonnaise
✦ Regular mayonnaise (use moderately—it is high in calories)
✦ Nonfat and reduced-fat salad dressings (compare labels for carb content)
✦ Regular salad dressings (use moderately—they are high in calories; choose brands made with canola, olive, soybean, or walnut oil)

Margarine and Butter

Like full-fat mayonnaise and salad dressing, margarine and butter can bust your calorie budget in a hurry. In addition, butter is loaded with artery-clogging saturated fat, and many brands of margarine contain harmful trans fat. The best advice is to use both sparingly. Light margarine and butter are widely available and work well for spreading on foods and in some cooking applications. Many brands of trans-free margarine are now available and are superior choices to margarines made with hydrogenated vegetable oils.

✦ Trans-free light margarine
✦ Trans-free regular margarine (use sparingly—it is high in calories)
✦ Light butter
✦ Regular butter (use sparingly—it is high in saturated fat and calories)
✦ Low-calorie buttery spray

Where Does Fat Fit In?

When eating a lower-carb diet, you can be a little more generous with your fat allowance. In fact, eating some fat may actually increase your chances for success because it makes food taste better and helps you feel satisfied. However, a high-fat free-for-all of bacon, cheese, butter, and pork rinds is taking things way too far!

As you plan your lower-carb meals, be mindful that fat is a very concentrated source of calories, so high-fat foods like fatty meats and cheeses, margarine, butter, salad dressings, olive oil, and nuts can slow weight loss—or even cause weight gain—if eaten in excess of your calorie needs. Furthermore, all fats are not created equal. The following inset explains why, and the recommendations in this chapter will help you choose the best fats to promote excellent health.

Good versus Bad Fats

Just as all carbohydrates are not created equal, neither are all fats. And while terms like saturated, trans, monos and polys, omega-3, and omega-6 can be mind-boggling, sorting the good fats from the bad is not as hard as most people think. Here are the basics of what you should know about dietary fats.

Saturated Fat

Saturated fats top the list of fats to avoid because they elevate LDL (bad) blood cholesterol levels and raise the risk for cardiovascular disease. Diets high in saturated fat are also associated with insulin resistance and a higher diabetes risk. Since fatty meats and dairy products are the main sources of saturated fat in most people's diets, you can easily trim your intake of this undesirable fat by choosing lean meats and low-fat dairy products. Coconuts, coconut oil, and palm kernel oil are also high in saturated fat, so foods containing these ingredients should be limited as well.

Trans Fat

This fat is formed when liquid vegetable oils are hydrogenated to make them more solid. Trans fats behave like saturated fats in the body, and may in fact be even worse for your health. Like saturated fats, trans fats raise LDL (bad) cholesterol. In addition, they lower HDL (good) cholesterol, posing a dual risk for cardiovascular disease. Diets high in trans fat have also been linked to insulin resistance and diabetes.

Trans fats are found in partially hydrogenated vegetable oils, vegetable shortenings, and hard margarines. Commercial bakery items, processed snack foods, fried foods, and other foods that contain shortening or hydrogenated vegetable oils are also big offenders.

Monounsaturated Fat

Popularized by the heart-healthy "Mediterranean diet," monounsaturated fats have become a staple in many people's diets. Olive oil is the best-known source of monounsaturated fat, but canola oil, avocadoes, and most nuts are rich in monounsaturated fats as well. While monounsaturated fats are a healthful choice, remember that they are still a concentrated source of calories, so include them in your diet with your weight-management goals in mind.

Polyunsaturated Fat

Two types of polyunsaturated fats, known as *omega-6* and *omega-3,* are essential for life. The ratio of these two fatty acids in your diet is also important because they have very powerful and very opposing effects in the body. Researchers believe that humans evolved on a diet that provided about equal amounts of omega-6 and omega-3 fats. Modern diets, however, which are based on grain-fed meats and hydrogenated oils, supply up to 20 times as much omega-6 as omega-3 fat. This imbalance favors the development of cardiovascular disease and may also promote cancer, inflammatory diseases like rheumatoid arthritis, and autoimmune disorders like lupus.

How can you get more omega-3 fats? Fatty fish is the best source of some especially potent omega-3 fats known as EPA and DHA. Among plant foods, flaxseeds and flax oil are the most concentrated sources. Canola oil, walnuts, and soy are also good sources of this essential fat.

COOKING OILS

Frequently referred to as "good fats," vegetable oils contain no carbs, are cholesterol-free, and are low in artery-clogging saturated fat. Unfortunately, many people are under the impression that they are also low in calories and can be used liberally in a low-carb diet. Nothing could be further from the truth. Since all oils are pure fat, they provide 120 calories per tablespoon. Use too much, and your weight loss may suffer.

On the other hand, using some oil (or other fat) in recipes can make food more palatable and satisfying, so there's no need to completely eliminate it. Moreover, some oils provide essential fats, such as the omega-3 fat alpha-linolenic acid that many people do not get enough of. Used wisely, cooking oils can enhance flavor and help provide a healthy balance of essential fat. Here are some of the better choices.

- Canola oil (good source of omega-3 fat)
- Extra-virgin olive oil
- Sesame oil
- Soybean oil (good source of omega-3 fat)
- Walnut oil (good source of omega-3 fat)
- Nonstick vegetable oil cooking sprays

CONDIMENTS AND SEASONINGS

A variety of herbs, spices, condiments, and seasonings can quickly change a dish from ordinary to extraordinary, greatly enhancing your dining pleasure.

- Anchovies and anchovy paste
- Capers
- Horseradish
- Hot sauce
- Lemon juice
- Mustard
- Pesto
- Salsa and picante sauce

A Simple Way to Lower the Glycemic Index of Meals

The naturally occurring acids in fruits, as well as the acids in fermented foods like yogurt and buttermilk, slow the rate at which these foods are digested and absorbed, and contribute to their low glycemic index. Likewise, adding just 4 teaspoons of vinegar or lemon juice to a meal can lower the GI of a meal by up to 30 percent. For this reason, using vinegar and lemon juice to flavor foods can be a simple but powerful way to lower the GI of your diet.

◆ Soy sauce (reduced-sodium)
◆ Spice blends such as Italian seasoning; fines herbes; herbes de Provence; curry paste (curry spices mixed with canola oil, ground lentils, and other ingredients); Mrs. Dash; lemon pepper; Cajun, Greek, and jerk seasonings
◆ Vinegars—apple cider, balsamic, champagne, malt, raspberry, sherry, rice, white, red wine, white wine, and others
◆ Worcestershire sauce
◆ Ketchup and barbecue sauce (lower-carb versions are now available in grocery stores.)
◆ Jams and preserves (for the Good-Carb Life Plan); choose low-sugar and all-fruit types

SNACK FOODS

Your snack choices can make or break your chances of weight-loss success. Unfortunately, in our "grab-and-go" society, foods like chips, pretzels, crackers, cereal bars, cookies, and sugary sodas top the list of popular snack foods. Loaded with refined carbs and low in fiber and nutrients, these products can wreak havoc on your blood sugar and actually trigger hunger and a vicious cycle of overeating.

What should you snack on instead? Try having some *real* food—a half sand-

Flavorful Spice Rubs

Herb and spice rubs are a simple way to perk up the flavor of meats, seafood, and poultry. A wide variety of blends are available in grocery stores today, but many contain added sugar and far too much salt. Here are some reduced-sodium, sugar-free recipes for your cooking pleasure. Each recipe makes about ⅓ cup. Store leftovers in an airtight container.

How to use: Rub over the surface of the meat, seafood, or poultry, using 3 to 4 teaspoons per pound. Grill, broil, sauté, or roast as desired.

Caribbean Spice Rub
Combine 1 tablespoon each ground paprika, dried thyme, lemon pepper, and onion powder with 2 teaspoons garlic powder, 1 teaspoon ground allspice, and 1 teaspoon salt.

Greek Spice Rub
Combine 1 tablespoon each dried oregano, rosemary, lemon pepper, and onion powder with 2 teaspoons garlic powder and 1 teaspoon salt.

Cajun Spice Rub
Combine 2 tablespoons ground paprika with 1 tablespoon onion powder, 2 teaspoons garlic powder, and 1 teaspoon each dried thyme, oregano, ground black pepper, and salt.

Southwestern Spice Rub
Combine 1 tablespoon each ground cumin, chili powder, dried oregano, and onion powder with 2 teaspoons garlic powder, ¾ teaspoon ground black pepper, and 1 teaspoon salt.

wich, hard-boiled egg, cup of soup, peanut butter on a celery stalk, apple with low-fat cheese, or leftovers from a previous meal. The following is a list of some additional snack items to stock up on. The menus in Chapter 4 provide more ideas for putting together wholesome and satisfying snacks.

- ✦ Low-fat string cheese
- ✦ Sugar-free yogurt
- ✦ Low-fat cottage cheese singles
- ✦ Roast turkey (or other lean meat) slices
- ✦ Fresh precut vegetables
- ✦ Single-serving cans of low-sodium vegetable or tomato juice
- ✦ Nuts and seeds (in moderation)
- ✦ Fresh fruit (for Good-Carb Life Plan)
- ✦ Light microwave popcorn (for Good-Carb Life Plan)

PROTEIN BARS AND SHAKES

Considered by many to be a convenient snack or meal on the go, protein bars and shakes have soared in popularity. But are these products all they're cracked up to be? Not always. In fact, many bars and shakes are little more than glorified junk food. There have even been cases in which protein bars were found to be mislabeled and to contain much more carbohydrate than the label stated.

Another problem with many protein bars and shakes is that they contain large amounts of added vitamins and minerals, which can be a problem if consumed in excess. Most of these products are also highly processed, so they lack the balance of naturally occurring nutrients and phytochemicals that are present in whole foods.

What about calories? Many protein bars and shakes are quite high in calories, considering their small serving size. In comparison, for the 200 or more calories contained in a typical protein bar, you could have half of a whole-wheat pita stuffed with 2 ounces of turkey, ¾ ounce of light Swiss cheese, and plenty of veggie trimmings!

On the other hand, some protein bars do pack in a substantial amount of protein (15 to 30 grams) with a minimum of questionable ingredients, and can fit the bill when you have limited access to "real" food. Just be sure to read labels carefully when choosing protein bars and shakes. Avoid those that are high in calories, artificial ingredients, or hydrogenated fats, or are overly fortified with nutrients and herbal supplements. Chosen wisely, protein bars and shakes can serve as an occasional substitute for meals and snacks, but don't let them replace too much of the real food in your diet.

PROTEIN POWDERS

Unlike protein bars and shakes, most protein powders are pure protein isolated from milk (whey), eggs (albumin), or soy. Protein powders can be a useful supplement for people who choose to avoid meat. Most products are fat-free and contain only a few grams of carbohydrate per serving.

How do you use protein powders? The most popular way is to add a scoop to your own fresh ingredients, to create a protein-rich smoothie or shake. Protein powder is typically less expensive than protein bars and shakes, making it a smart addition to the low-carb pantry. Each type of protein powder has a slightly different flavor, so experiment and see which you prefer.

SWEETS AND DESSERTS

Satisfying the sweet tooth can be a real challenge when cutting carbs. Here are some lower-carb products to enjoy when on the Good-Carb Life Plan. You should be aware that "sugar-free" and "low-carb" products may or may not be lower in calories than the "real thing," so always compare calories before buying. Chapter 15 also presents an assortment of lighter options for dessert.

*   Sugar-free pudding mixes
*   Sugar-free gelatin
*   Sugar-free Fudgesicles
*   Sugar-free Popsicles
*   100 percent fruit and juice bars
*   Fruits canned in natural juice
*   Unsweetened applesauce
*   Low-fat or light (no added sugar) ice cream and frozen yogurt (see the inset on page 251 for more on choosing ice cream)
*   Dark chocolate (high in calories, use in moderation)

Is Sugar-Free All It's Cracked Up to Be?

As the pendulum swings back to a lower-carb, sugar-busting mindset, so do products offered by manufacturers. Grocery stores now offer a plethora of "sugar-free" cookies, candies, ice cream, and other confections. But is sugar-free really any better than the real thing? Not always.

People are often surprised to find that some sugar-free products have just as many calories as the products they are meant to replace. (This is why many of these products bear labels that state "Not For Weight Control.") How can this be? For one thing, extra fat is frequently added to make up for the flavor and texture that is lost when sugar is removed. In addition, most sugar-free cookies and baked goods still contain a high proportion of white flour, which adds carbs and calories.

What gives sugar-free products their sweetness? Many products contain "sugar alcohols" such as maltitol, sorbitol, and hydrogenated starch hydrolysates. These carbohydrate-based sweeteners are incompletely absorbed by the body, so they provide about half the calories of sugar and they have a milder effect on blood glucose and insulin levels. However, as mentioned above, other ingredients like flour and fat still add calories, so the net calorie reduction in sugar-free food may not be as much as you might expect.

Be aware, too, that sugar alcohols can cause bloating, gas, and have a laxative effect if too much is eaten. On the other hand, sweeteners like aspartame (NutraSweet, or Equal), saccharine (Sweet'n Low), acesulfame-K (Sunett), and sucralose (Splenda) do not add a significant number of calories to foods or cause a laxative effect. (For more on sugar substitutes, see pages 81–83.)

Chosen carefully, you will find that some sugar-free products—like sodas, gelatin, pudding, yogurt, hot cocoa mix, and some brands of frozen Fudgesicles and juice bars—can be a real boon to the carb-conscious person. On the other hand, sugar-free cookies, cakes, and candies often save few or no calories and may still be quite high in carbohydrate. The bottom line is that you should always read labels—and first and foremost, compare calories if you are watching your weight.

+ Sugar-free chocolate milk
+ Sugar-free hot chocolate
+ Light (sugar-free or low-sugar) pie fillings
+ Sugar-free strawberry glaze for making pies and desserts
+ Nonfat and light whipped toppings
+ Oatmeal cookies made with nonhydrogenated fats (high in carbs, so eat in moderation)

BAKING INGREDIENTS

On the Good-Carb Life Plan, you can enjoy a variety of wholesome home-made baked goods as well as an occasional sweet treat. The following ingredients will help you create treats that are both healthful and delicious. To prevent rancidity, be sure to store whole-grain flours, flaxmeal, and wheat germ in the refrigerator or freezer.

+ Flaxseeds—Loaded with healthful omega-3 fats, flaxseeds can be ground in a blender or coffee grinder into flaxmeal, which can replace 10 to 25 percent of the flour in muffins, quick breads, and other recipes. (Note: Flax experts recommend limiting intake to 1 tablespoon of ground flaxseed per day until more is known about the health effects of consuming larger amounts.)
+ Rolled oats and oat bran—Replace part of the flour in muffins, quick breads, and other recipes with oatmeal or oat bran for a fiber and nutrition boost.
+ Oat flour—Ground from whole-grain oats, oat flour lends a slightly sweet flavor and a tender texture to baked goods, reducing the need for fat and sugar. Rich in fiber and nutrients, oat flour also improves the nutritional profile of foods when you substitute it for part of the white flour in recipes. These qualities make oat flour a natural for healthy baking. Oat flour can replace up to half of the flour in products like muffins, quick breads, cakes, and cookies. You can purchase oat flour in natural food stores and in some grocery stores. Or make your own by grinding quick-cooking oats in a blender or food processor. One cup of oats yields about ¾ cup of flour.

- ✦ Wheat bran—Give a fiber boost to muffins and quick breads by replacing part of the flour with wheat bran.
- ✦ Wheat germ—Loaded with vitamin E, minerals, and B vitamins. Replace up to 25 percent of the flour in baked goods with this super-nutritious product.
- ✦ Whole-wheat flour—Use to replace part or all of the white flour in homemade yeast breads.
- ✦ White whole-wheat flour—A lighter-tasting alternative to regular whole-wheat flour. This product can be used in yeast breads and quick breads, muffins, pancakes, and many other recipes.
- ✦ Whole-wheat pastry flour—Made especially for products like muffins, quick breads, cookies, and pancakes, this product has a lightly sweet flavor and softer texture than regular whole-wheat flour.

SUGAR SUBSTITUTES

In a quest to trim carbs and calories from recipes, many people turn to sugar substitutes. However, when using these products in recipes, it's important to understand that sugar adds more than just sweetness. For instance, sugar adds texture and tenderness, helps retain moisture, and promotes the browning of baked goods. For this reason, replacing all of the sugar in foods like cakes, cookies, and muffins with a sugar substitute can result in a very disappointing (pale, rubbery, and dry) product. This is why some of the recipes in this book do contain some real sugar. On the other hand, products like pies, fruit crisps, puddings, and gelatin desserts more easily adapt to using sugar substitutes. A wide variety of sugar substitutes is available to choose from. Here is a brief description of some of these products and their suitability for recipes.

Acesulfame-K
Sold under the brand name Sunett, acesulfame-K has a pleasant flavor and leaves no bitter aftertaste. This product is heat stable, so it can be used in cooked foods.

Aspartame
Also known as NutraSweet or Equal, aspartame is made of two amino acids (the building blocks of proteins). It has a pleasant flavor and leaves no bitter af-

What Are "Net Carbs"?

Anyone who adopts a low-carb diet will soon hear terms like "net carbs," "effective carbs," or "digestible carbs." These terms, which are used interchangeably, are calculated by subtracting all of the dietary fiber and sugar alcohols from the total carbohydrate content of a food. For instance, a protein bar that contains 22 grams of carbohydrate, 18 grams of sugar alcohol, and 2 grams of fiber, would have only 2 net carbs. How valid is this rationale?

It's very reasonable to subtract all of the fiber from the carbohydrate count on a food label. This is because dietary fiber is included in the total carbohydrate amount listed on the label, but is not digested or absorbed—so it has no impact on blood sugar levels and provides no calories.

Like fiber, sugar alcohols are included in the total carbohydrate amount listed on food labels. These sweeteners are not completely digested and absorbed, so they provide about half the calories as white table sugar and they have a much gentler impact on blood sugar levels. A point of contention, though, is whether it's valid to subtract *all* of the sugar alcohols from the carbohydrate content of a food, as is done with fiber. Because sugar alcohols do provide some calories and have a small impact on blood sugar, it's probably more reasonable to subtract only half of the sugar alcohols from the total carbs listed on the label.

Is all this math really necessary when choosing foods? Definitely not. And there's a real danger in getting so caught up in carb counting that you forget to look at total calories, fat, and other nutritional attributes of a food. The tips, menus, and recipes featured throughout this book will help you choose the best carbs for lifelong health and long-term weight control.

tertaste. Aspartame can be used in some cooked and baked recipes, but may lose its sweetness if cooked for too long or at temperatures that are too high. This is why it's best to add this sweetener at the end of the cooking process whenever possible. One of the amino acids in aspartame, phenylalanine, must be avoided by people who have a genetic disorder known as phenylketonuria (PKU). People who have this disorder cannot break down phenylalanine, so it accumulates in their blood, resulting in neurological problems. This is why aspartame-containing products are labeled with a warning to this effect.

Saccharin

For many years, saccharin (sold under the brand name Sweet'n Low) was sold with a warning that it caused cancer in laboratory animals. In 2000, this warning was discontinued as the FDA determined saccharin to be safe for human consumption. Saccharin is heat stable and may be used in cooking, but used in large amounts, it has a bitter aftertaste.

Sucralose

Sold under the brand name Splenda, this sweetener is made from sucrose, through a process that substitutes chlorine atoms for part of the sugar molecule. Sucralose has a natural sugar flavor with no bitter aftertaste. It is also is heat stable, so can be used for cooking and baking. Of the products currently available on the market, sucralose is, by far, the best suited for cooking and baking.

Stevia

This herbal sweetener has been used in South America for centuries. It has also been used in Japan since the early 1970s. Some brands of Stevia have a slight licoricelike flavor that people might find overpowering. While stevia has no known adverse effects, it has not yet been approved by the FDA for use as a sweetener, which is why you won't find stevia sold alongside other sweeteners in your grocery store. You can, however, buy stevia in health-food stores, where it is sold as a dietary supplement. Realize that dietary supplements are not regulated as stringently as FDA-approved food ingredients, and may have no guarantees of purity or long-term safety.

SUGAR AND OTHER
CALORIC SWEETENERS

While cutting back on sugar is an important part of your low-carb lifestyle, there's no need to go to extremes. As previously mentioned, some recipes just aren't the same without a bit of real sugar. And completely depriving yourself of sugar might just make you crave it more. If you opt to begin with the Low-Carb Quick-Start Plan, you will temporarily give up sugar. But once you progress to the Good-Carb Life Plan, you will find that small amounts of sugar (and other sweeteners, like honey, maple syrup, molasses, and brown sugar) *can* be included in a healthy eating plan. The menus and recipes in this book provide many examples of how to keep sugar in perspective.

6.

Eating Well When You're Away from Home

Most people find that controlling carbs is easily mastered at home, where they have maximal control over food choices. But can you maintain your carb-conscious lifestyle in restaurants, at work, and on the road? Absolutely. This chapter presents a wealth of ideas for eating well regardless of your setting or situation.

Whether you're grabbing a fast-food meal, eating breakfast at the local diner, or enjoying dinner at a fine restaurant, you'll find that many appealing options are there for the taking. There are also plenty of tricks for eating smart at the office and on the road. It's even possible to enjoy a holiday party without blowing your carb or calorie budgets, or turn a cocktail party into a satisfying *dinner* party. As you will see, a good carb/low-carb lifestyle can be both enjoyable and easy to implement—anywhere, anytime, and anyplace.

DILEMMAS OF DINING OUT

Since more than half of all Americans eat out on any given day, our away-from-home food choices can have a big impact on our overall diet. The problem is that this impact is usually a lot more negative than positive—since most people end up eating far more calories, fat, and carbs in restaurants than they would at home. Does this mean you should just give up and eat at home all the time? Definitely not. Any eating plan that forces you to become a social recluse will never stand the test of time. Besides, a wide variety of delicious lower-carb meals can be enjoyed in just about any restaurant.

THE RESTAURANT REVOLUTION

In recent years, the restaurant industry has become acutely aware that a majority of their customers are watching their weight or dealing with health problems like insulin resistance, prediabetes, and diabetes. Realizing that it's good business to give customers what they want, most are more than willing to let you "have it your way." Some restaurants even offer special meals that fit perfectly into a healthful lower-carb eating plan. Following are some general guidelines for dining defensively in any restaurant.

Breakfast

If you are following the Low-Carb Quick-Start Plan, you will be temporarily limited to breakfast foods like bacon, sausage, and eggs. However, to avoid an overdose of saturated fat, ask for Canadian bacon or ham, which is much leaner than regular bacon and sausage. Many restaurants also offer fat-free egg substitutes, like Egg Beaters, and can whip you up a delicious omelet filled with plenty of veggies and a sprinkling of cheese. If the restaurant does not offer egg substitutes, see if they will make your omelet with more whites and fewer yolks. When dining in a vegetarian restaurant, you may also find dishes like scrambled eggs with tofu accompanied by vegetarian sausage or bacon. Other menu items that are compatible with the Quick-Start Plan include cottage cheese, tomato juice, V-8 juice, and low-fat milk.

On the Good-Carb Life Plan, your choices are much more varied. Add a dish of fresh fruit to your low-fat omelet, or have a poached egg on a piece of whole-wheat toast. A steaming bowl of oatmeal or a cold, high-fiber cereal with low-fat milk is another good choice. In the mood for French toast? Ask to have it made with whole-wheat bread and topped with fresh fruit. Some restaurants also offer sugar-free or light syrup.

Appetizers

Best bets include steamed or grilled seafood, such as shrimp, mussels, or oysters; tomato juice or a Virgin Mary; broth-based vegetable soups and bean soups; and salads with a small amount of dressing (avoid sweet dressings like honey-mustard and French).

Entrées

Just about every restaurant offers a delectable selection of worthy entrées—including skinless chicken, fish and shellfish, sirloin and filet mignon steaks, and pork tenderloin. As for preparation methods, choose from broiled, blackened, grilled, pan-seared, stir-fried, poached, baked, roasted, and en papillote (steamed in parchment paper). Steer clear of fatty sauces like hollandaise and béarnaise, and instead choose entrées served au jus, or accompanied by wine, broth, or tomato-based sauces.

Side Dishes

Side dishes can make or break your carb-conscious eating plan, so avoid the rice and potatoes and opt instead for a double portion of veggies. Most restaurants feature a "vegetable of the day" such as a sautéed vegetable medley, green beans with almonds, or steamed broccoli and cauliflower. Other excellent choices include sautéed mushrooms and roasted or grilled vegetable combinations.

Main-Dish Salads

From fine dining to fast food, a glorious main-dish salad can be had in just about any restaurant. Choose salads topped with nonfried chicken or seafood, turkey, lean ham, or other lean protein, and plenty of extra veggies. Use just a couple of tablespoons of dressing instead of the 4 to 6 tablespoons that typically come with the salad. Keep the cheese to a light sprinkling, since most restaurants use the full-fat kind. Avoid "edible" shells such as fried tortilla bowls, and omit starchy toppings like croutons, fried rice noodles, and tortilla strips. Instead, add a light sprinkling of nuts or sunflower seeds for added crunch.

Sandwiches

Made properly, a hearty sandwich can be a perfect fit for your Good-Carb Life Plan program. Just be sure to request whole-grain bread, and avoid sandwiches made with extra-thick bread slices or supersize buns and rolls. Choose turkey, grilled chicken, lean roast beef, or other lean protein as a filling, and pile on plenty of veggie toppings. Request mustard, light mayo, or light ranch dressing as a spread instead of full-fat mayo and "special sauces." Avoid a carbohydrate overload by pairing your sandwich with a cup of vegetable soup, a salad, fresh fruit, or cottage cheese instead of chips or pretzels.

Dessert

On the Good-Carb Life Plan, dessert is not necessarily out of the question—just make it the exception instead of the rule. When you do have dessert, your best bet is to get what you really want and split it with someone—or several others. That way you still get most of the enjoyment but a lot less calories.

STEERING CLEAR OF TEMPTATION

While most restaurants will happily cater to your requests for healthful eating, they also cater to tastes for excess and overindulgence—and steering clear of temptation can be difficult at times. Here are some tips to help you avoid diet disasters.

✦ Don't starve yourself all day in anticipation of having dinner out. This will cause your blood sugar to dip so low that once you start eating, you won't be able to stop until you've really overdone it.

✦ Check out the menu before you go. Many restaurants feature their menus online, allowing you to determine your options well in advance.

✦ Pass up the bread basket. The same goes for the tortilla chips served in Tex-Mex restaurants. Ask your server to leave it in the kitchen, or at the very least, put it on the far side of the table if your dinner companions are not cutting carbs.

✦ Beware of buffets. An excellent low-carb meal can be had from the buffet line, but if passing up so many high-carb and high-calorie choices leaves you feeling deprived, it's best to pass on the buffet and choose a restaurant that offers table service.

✦ Beware of portion distortion. Restaurants have led the way in the supersizing trend. Since many restaurants provide enough food for two meals, take half home and get two meals for the price of one. Alternatively, split an entrée with a dinner companion or ask if they will serve a lunch-size portion at dinner. Some restaurants also offer "light" (smaller) portions at a reduced price.

MASTERING THE MENU

Each type of restaurant poses its own challenges and rewards, but with just a little insight and creativity, you can easily enjoy a healthful and delicious meal at just about any establishment. Here are some tips for making the most of the menu in a variety of settings. (Note that the higher-carb dishes listed below should be reserved for the Good-Carb Life Plan regimen.) The menus in Chapter 4 provide more ideas for including restaurant fare in your low-carb meal plans.

Restaurant Type	*Menu Suggestions*
CHINESE	✦ Broth-based soups like hot and sour and egg drop ✦ Stir-fried combinations of seafood, poultry, lean meat, tofu, and vegetables ✦ Steamed fish and vegetable dishes ✦ Szechuan sauce, bean sauce, shrimp sauce, oyster sauce, hot mustard ✦ Moderate portion of steamed brown rice, if available (for Good-Carb Life Plan only)
FRENCH	✦ Consommé and broth-based soups, mussels (steamed or cooked in a tomato-wine sauce) ✦ Broiled, steamed, or poached seafood and poultry (order sauces on the side) ✦ Seafood and poultry cooked en papillote (steamed in parchment paper) ✦ Chicken or fish Provençal (with tomato sauce), chicken or fish cooked with tomato-wine sauces ✦ Coq au vin (chicken braised in wine sauce) ✦ Seafood or vegetable stews, such as bouillabaisse and ratatouille ✦ Chicken and beef stews with wine or tomato sauces

FRENCH (continued)	✦ Steamed or roasted vegetables ✦ Salads with dressing on the side
GREEK	✦ Bean and lentil soups, vegetable soups, fish soups ✦ Souvlaki (shish kebabs) of chicken, lean beef or pork, or roasted lamb, and vegetables ✦ Baked fish dishes such as plaki (fish baked with tomatoes, onions, and garlic) and fish baked in grape leaves ✦ Baked chicken dishes ✦ Salads topped with a light sprinkling of feta cheese and vinaigrette dressing on the side
INDIAN	✦ Vegetable and dal (lentil or bean) soups ✦ Vegetable, seafood, and chicken curry dishes (avoid those made with large amounts of coconut or coconut milk) ✦ Chicken or shrimp vindaloo (in a hot and spicy tomato, onion, and curry sauce; may contain potatoes); (for Good-Carb Life Plan only) ✦ Tandoori chicken or fish (chicken or fish marinated in yogurt and spices and baked in a clay oven) ✦ Lamb or chicken kebabs ✦ Raita (a cold side dish made of cucumbers or other vegetables with yogurt sauce) ✦ Chutney (a spicy accompaniment to meals)
ITALIAN	✦ Vegetable or bean-based soups like white bean and escarole, minestrone, and pasta fagioli ✦ Steamed clams or mussels ✦ Insalata frutti de mare (seafood salad) ✦ Broiled or grilled chicken and fish dishes ✦ Chicken cacciatore, piccata, and marsala ✦ Seafood stews like cioppino ✦ Moderate portions of pasta with tomato sauces like marinara, puttanesca, and arrabbiata; pasta with tomato-seafood sauce like red clam sauce (for Good-Carb Life Plan only); (ask if half- or lunch-size portions are available at dinner)

ITALIAN *(continued)*	✦ Thin-crust pizza with vegetable toppings (for Good-Carb Life Plan only); (add a side salad for nutritional balance) ✦ Cappuccino made with low-fat milk
JAPANESE	✦ Miso soup, broth-based soup ✦ Yakitori (broiled chicken kebabs), teriyaki dishes, yaki-mono (grilled) dishes, sukiyaki (thinly sliced beef and vegetables in a piquant sauce) ✦ Stir-fried seafood, chicken, lean beef, or tofu and vegetable combinations ✦ Moderate portions of whole-wheat udon noodles, buckwheat soba noodles, rice noodles, and steamed brown rice (for Good-Carb Life Plan) ✦ Wasabi (Japanese horseradish)
MEXICAN	✦ Black-bean soup, ceviche (lime-marinated seafood salad), gazpacho (chilled tomato and cucumber soup) ✦ Grilled fish and chicken dishes ✦ Salsa, tomatillo sauce, verde (green) sauce, pico de gallo (tomatoes with onions and hot peppers) ✦ Guacamole (in moderation—it is high in calories) ✦ Chicken soft tacos and burritos (for Good-Carb Life Plan only). Note: when choosing tortilla-based entrées, avoid those made with supersize tortilla wraps and rice fillings. Also, see if whole-wheat tortillas are available, and limit the high-fat cheese and sour cream. ✦ Chicken, shrimp, and vegetable fajitas (for Good-Carb Life Plan only); (see if whole-wheat tortillas are available, and limit the sour cream and cheese toppings)
THAI	✦ Broth-based soups like tom yum gai (chicken with vegetables and Thai seasonings) or tom yum goong (shrimp with vegetables and Thai seasonings) ✦ Stir-fried combinations of seafood, chicken, tofu, lean meat, and vegetables ✦ *Moderate* portions of pad Thai and other stir-fried noodle dishes made with vegetables and seafood, chicken, tofu, or lean meat (for Good-Carb Life Plan only)

THAI *(continued)*	✦ Dishes made with basil sauce, lime sauce, chili sauce, fish sauce
STEAK HOUSES	✦ Shish kebabs ✦ Small sirloin or tenderloin (filet mignon) steaks ✦ Grilled skinless chicken and seafood ✦ Grilled steak or chicken salads with light dressing (limit cheese and bacon toppings) ✦ Side salad with light dressing; steamed or grilled vegetables ✦ Baked sweet potatoes (for Good-Carb Life Plan only)
DELIS AND SUB SHOPS	✦ Salads topped with turkey, lean roast beef, or other lean meats with light dressing ✦ Vegetable and bean soups ✦ Turkey or lean meat sandwiches or 6-inch subs on whole-grain bread with plenty of vegetable toppings (for Good-Carb Life Plan only) ✦ Whole-wheat wraps filled with turkey or lean meat and vegetables (for Good-Carb Life Plan only)
FAST FOOD	✦ Grilled chicken salads with light dressing ✦ Chili and side salad ✦ Grilled chicken sandwiches on multigrain bun spread with mustard, light mayo, or light ranch dressing (Good-Carb Life Plan only)

WORKDAY SURVIVAL

For millions of people, the workplace is a huge barrier to weight-loss success. This is especially true if your job involves sitting at a desk all day. Add a long commute, and you are left with almost no opportunity to be physically active. As if that's not bad enough, the workplace abounds with occupational eating hazards. From double mocha lattes and morning donuts to vending machines, desktop candy jars, treats brought in by coworkers, and lunches out, there are countless opportunities to overindulge during the workday. But what really tips the scale is workplace boredom and stress, which are often confused with

Coffee—Is It Out of Control?

Once a simple brew—served in an 8-ounce cup, black or with just a touch of cream and sugar—coffee has become an out-of-control supersize concoction laced with loads of sugar and covered with whipped cream. Made with whole milk and sugar, a large latte easily delivers 250 calories. Supersizing and adding ingredients like half-and-half, cream, whipped cream, and flavored syrups, can more than double the calories.

What to do? Get back to basics: Begin by choosing a smaller (8- to 12-ounce) serving. Lighten your beverage with nonfat or low-fat milk, and skip the sugar or use a sugar substitute. Instead of whipped cream, flavored syrup, and chocolate or candy toppings, embellish your brew with a sprinkle of cinnamon or cocoa powder.

hunger. Faced with this combination of circumstances, your resolve to eat well can easily crumble. How can you gain better control over your workday? Here are some suggestions.

✦　Eat a balanced breakfast that includes some protein and fiber. This will get your blood sugar on an even keel and set the tone for what you eat the rest of the day. You will be less likely to succumb to the junk food around you.

✦　Eat a balanced lunch—again with some protein and fiber. This will help prevent that mid-afternoon slump that sends people to the vending machine.

✦　Keep healthy snacks at work. If you have access to a refrigerator, that's the best-case scenario because most grab-and-go snack foods (like crackers, pretzels, and cookies) are loaded with refined carbs and lack protein. Instead, low-fat string cheese, single-serving containers of cottage cheese and sugar-free yogurt, a cup of low-fat milk, a small handful of nuts, a hard-boiled egg, and fresh raw vegetables are perfect for the Low-Carb Quick-Start. If you are on the Good-Carb Life Plan, add to this list snacks like half a sandwich on whole-grain bread, fresh fruit, single-serving con-

The Best Place for the Candy Jar

"Out of sight is out of mind" is just as true at work as it is at home. In a recent study, researchers evaluated where office workers kept their candy jars and how much candy they ate. They discovered that people who kept candy jars on their desktops ate three pieces more each day than people who stashed their candy out of sight in a desk drawer. Even more notable, people with desktop candy jars ate *six* pieces more each day than coworkers who had to walk six feet away from their desk to get candy. Of course, having no candy jar at all is the best-case scenario!

tainers of no-added-sugar fruit, unsweetened applesauce, and low-fat microwave popcorn.

✦ Request better choices in the vending machine, snack bar, and cafeteria.

✦ Request on-site exercise classes. More and more employers understand that fit and healthy employees keep company insurance costs down, reduce sick days, increase productivity, and improve profits. To help people stay well, many companies offer on-site gyms and/or exercise classes. Some even offer bonuses for people who exercise. It can be as simple as using a conference room for a Pilates or body-shaping class several times a week.

✦ Walk during your breaks at work. Even a few minutes outdoors will break the monotony, re-energize you, and reduce the desire to snack. Also, take the stairs instead of the elevator, and get up and stretch periodically. If possible, use your lunch hour to go to the gym, and then eat lunch at your desk.

✦ Enlist the support of coworkers and management to "detoxify" your work environment. Worksite weight gain is such a pervasive problem that your coworkers may welcome a more proactive environment. Start by getting rid of those desktop candy jars. Instead of celebrating birthdays with cake and ice cream, give out movie tickets or some other nonfood token of recognition. Serve fruit, sugar-free yogurt, low-fat cheese and milk, and bran muffins at morning meetings instead of pastries and donuts.

Taking Your Show on the Road

Whether you're traveling for work or pleasure, being out of town and away from your routine can quickly derail your healthy lifestyle. Here are some suggestions for making the most of life on the road.

- When traveling by car, consider packing a cooler stocked with yogurt, sandwich and salad fixings, and beverages. Then, weather permitting, find a rest stop and enjoy a picnic lunch instead of going to a restaurant. This will provide a nice break and a chance to walk and stretch as well.
- When flying to your destination, pack your own snacks to take onboard. Small packets of sunflower seeds or nuts, fruit, and protein bars travel well. Use a small insulated bag for items like low-fat string cheese, yogurt, and sandwiches. Avoid the pretzels that most airlines provide for a snack. Their high glycemic index can wreak havoc on your blood sugar and trigger hunger.
- If you have a long layover, there are plenty of good food choices available in airports these days. For a quick snack, you can almost always find a deli or coffee shop that sells cartons of sugar-free yogurt, fresh fruit cups, chef or grilled-chicken salads, soups, and lean-meat sandwiches on whole-grain bread. Major airports also have full-service restaurants, including some national chains that offer a variety of appropriate meals.
- Time permitting, walk to your departure gates instead of using the trams and moving sidewalks. If you have a long layover, walk around the airport.
- Take plenty of reading material, work, or handicrafts with you to fill long flights, layovers, and unexpected delays. Keeping busy is the best way to prevent eating out of boredom.
- Keep plenty of water handy so that you don't find yourself snacking when you're really just thirsty.

When You Get There

Once you get to your destination, here are some simple things you can do to stay on course.

◆ If your hotel has a breakfast buffet, choose items like fruit, low-fat milk, oatmeal, sugar-free yogurt, scrambled eggs, and Canadian bacon, if available.

◆ Stock up on healthy snacks at a local market so the minibar won't tempt you.

◆ Ask the hotel staff if there are parks or trails nearby where you can walk or hike.

◆ Take a walking tour of the city. Many cities have maps for just this purpose.

◆ Be sure to pack your workout clothes, as many hotels have workout facilities that offer both aerobic and weight machines. You can also pack equipment like a jump rope, exercise band, or resistance tube. Add some push-ups and crunches for a simple but well-rounded workout in the privacy of your room.

HANDLING HOLIDAYS AND SPECIAL OCCASIONS

If special occasions were few and far between, a once-in-awhile overindulgence would not be a problem. But when you add up all the holidays, birthdays, weddings, parties, and other social gatherings that crop up during the year, it's clear that the amount of food eaten at these events is no trivial matter. Besides, once you discover how delicious and enjoyable lower-carb living can be, and how great you look and feel on your slimmed-down diet, you'll want to eat this way all year round.

Preparing for the Party Circuit

Too often, food is the focus of social gatherings, and the pressure to eat can be enormous. The good news is that a little advance planning can go a long way toward helping you survive the party circuit.

◆ **Plan ahead.** If you know you will be going to a party, work it into your daily meal plan. Save a third to a fourth of your daily food intake for a cocktail party, and half to a third of your allotment for a dinner party.

◆ **Turn a cocktail party into "dinner."** Heavy hors d'oeuvres can and should be considered dinner for anyone who is watching his or her weight. That said, you can create a fairly balanced meal from most party spreads. Start with an entrée—steamed seafood is an excellent choice. From the cold-cut tray, select items like sliced turkey, lean roast beef, and ham. Moving on to the next course, pile on plenty of fresh veggies, limiting any fatty dips that accompany them. For dessert, savor a selection of fresh fruit with a few cubes of cheese and a small portion of nuts, if available.

✦ **Don't be afraid to indulge.** On occasion, have a small portion of something decadent that you really want. Enjoy it!

✦ **Position yourself strategically.** Make a conscious effort to position yourself away from the buffet or hors d'oeuvres table.

✦ **Use a small plate.** This will create the illusion that you are getting more food.

✦ **Choose low-calorie libations.** For instance, have wine or a wine spritzer (wine mixed with club soda and lime) instead of a sweet wine cooler. Have light beer instead of regular. Choose liquors combined with sugar-free mixers instead of creamy or sweet drinks. Of course, sparkling water or diet soda are your best bets.

✦ **Mix and mingle.** Place more emphasis on the social aspect of the gathering, rather than food and drink.

When It's Your Party

When you're the host, there's plenty you can do to offer food that is both healthful and delicious. For instance, lean meat and low-fat cheese trays, steamed seafood platters, smoked salmon, mini kebabs, assorted fresh vegetables with low-fat dip, fresh fruits with no-added-sugar yogurt or light sour-cream dip, and hummus and olivada or tapenade with wedges of whole-grain pita bread are all excellent choices for your get-togethers. Chapter 8 also presents a selection of tempting recipes for party-perfect treats.

✧✦✧✦✦

As you have seen, adopting a carb-conscious lifestyle need not cause a major disruption in your daily activities or mean becoming a social recluse. Whatever the situation—dining at your favorite restaurant, traveling for work or pleasure, or hitting the party circuit, you *can* eat well and stay on course with your healthy lifestyle goals.

7.

~~~~~~

The Exercise-Carbohydrate Connection

No discussion of good-carb/low-carb living would be complete without talking about exercise. There is no question that physical activity will help you meet your weight-loss and health goals faster and better. An active lifestyle is also absolutely essential for long-term weight maintenance.

People who are carbohydrate sensitive should also keep in mind that physical activity boosts the body's ability to process carbohydrate and helps reduce insulin resistance. This means that physically active people can include a higher proportion of carbohydrate in their daily diet than sedentary people can without suffering ill effects.

Exercise acts much like an "insulin-sensitizing" drug to make the body's cells more responsive to insulin, which enables them to remove sugar from the blood more efficiently. As a result, the pancreas does not have to secrete as much insulin to keep blood sugar under control, the body's insulin levels drop, and you become less insulin resistant.

Exercise also builds and strengthens muscles—the body's main "clearinghouse" for blood glucose. In fact, muscles account for about 75 percent of glucose disposal by the body. So maintaining a healthy proportion of lean body mass is key to revving up your body's capacity to process carbohydrate.

MANY REASONS TO GET MOVING

An improved ability to process dietary carbohydrate is just one reason to enjoy an active lifestyle. What other benefits might you expect? Most people quickly notice an increased energy level, less vulnerability to stress, and improved feelings of well-being. Within weeks their muscles begin to appear more toned and their clothes fit more loosely.

Regular exercise will also reduce your risk for cardiovascular disease, cancer, and diabetes. It builds stronger bones and reduces the risk of osteoporosis. Exercise has been found to improve memory and slow the age-related decline in mental function. It can improve sexual functioning, and it makes people feel better about their bodies. There is no drug or magic pill that even comes close to matching the power of physical activity.

EXERCISE AND YOUR WEIGHT

Many health benefits can be derived from being active for just thirty minutes on most days of the week. However, this is not enough to prevent the "creeping weight gain" syndrome in most people. How much is enough to keep weight in check? People who lose weight and keep it off long-term accumulate about an hour of physical activity daily.

Where will you find the time to squeeze an hour of exercise into an already full day? It's easier than you may think, since your hour of physical activity can be done all at once or divided into several smaller bouts. This provides plenty of options to be flexible and creative. Everyday activities like vigorous house- and yard work, washing the car, and walking your dog can all count. The important thing is to just get moving, and keep in mind that *any exercise is better than none at all*.

It's imperative to choose practical and enjoyable activities so that your exercise program does not become just another chore. For instance, socialize with a friend over a walk, bike ride, or canoe trip instead of dinner and a movie. Plant a vegetable or flower garden, or take a family hike. Take the stairs instead of the elevator. Walk to lunch. It all adds up.

Making the Most of Your Exercise Program

Your exercise program can be as simple or elaborate as you want. As you have seen, by consciously squeezing in a few minutes of activity here and there during your daily routine, and by substituting active leisure-time hobbies for part of your television and computer time, you *can* meet the goal of being active for an hour a day.

What about different *types* of exercises—are some better than others? A well-rounded exercise program includes activities that strengthen both your cardiovascular system *and* your muscles. With a little forethought and creativity, you can plan your activities to target each of these areas, and derive maximal weight-loss and health benefits.

Aerobic Exercise

Aerobic exercise encompasses low- to moderate-intensity activities such as brisk walking, jogging, biking, racquet sports, swimming, and dancing. Activities like raking leaves, using a push mower, and mopping the floor can also be considered aerobic exercise. These forms of exercise are fueled mostly by fat, which can be burned only when there is plenty of oxygen present in the exercising muscles.

Because aerobic exercise forces the body to use increased amounts of oxygen, it makes the heart and lungs work harder and strengthens the cardiovascular system. As you become more aerobically fit, your muscles will become more sensitive to insulin and better able to remove sugar from the blood, reducing the risk for diabetes. Your muscles will also develop more fat-burning enzymes and become more efficient at burning fat both during exercise and while at rest.

Try to engage in some form of aerobic activity for at least thirty minutes on most days of the week. If you can squeeze in forty-five to sixty minutes, that would be even better. And don't forget that you can divide your activity sessions into several smaller bouts throughout the day.

Simple Ways to Become More Active

Being active does not necessarily mean going to the gym or joining a formal exercise class. And the little things you do day in and day out can have a tremendous impact over time. Here are some simple ways to add activity to your daily routine.

✦ Make exercise a social event—meet up with a friend for a walk or a game of tennis.

✦ Play basketball with your kids.

✦ Take a short walk during your breaks at work.

✦ Take the stairs instead of the elevator or escalator.

✦ Park farther away when you go shopping and run errands.

✦ Get off the subway or bus a stop earlier and walk to your destination.

✦ Enjoy walks with your dog.

✦ View household chores like cleaning, raking leaves, mowing the yard, shoveling snow, chopping firewood, and washing the car as opportunities to be more active.

✦ Plan a hike or biking excursion with family or friends.

✦ Exercise while watching television.

✦ While watching television, get up during commercial breaks and make the bed, load the dishwasher, etc. Lose the remote control.

✦ Plant a vegetable, herb, or flower garden.

✦ Wear a pedometer to track the number of steps you take in a day. (Two-thousand steps is the equivalent of 1 mile, and burns about 100 calories.)

✦ Instead of lying around the pool, jump in and do some laps or pool exercises.

Television and Your Weight

Everyone knows that sitting around watching television can cause weight gain. But a recent study demonstrated just how dangerous this habit can be. Researchers who tracked the television-viewing habits of more than 50,000 women discovered that each two-hour increment of daily TV time raised the risk of obesity by 23 percent. On the other hand, an hour a day of brisk walking reduced the risk of obesity by 24 percent. The researchers calculated that simply limiting TV time to less than ten hours per week and taking a brisk walk for thirty minutes per day could prevent 30 percent of new cases of obesity.

STRENGTH TRAINING

Strength training is any exercise that builds and strengthens muscles. Activities that build muscles include weight lifting, calisthenics (like push-ups and pull-ups), and body-shaping classes that use free weights or resistance tubes. Activities like chopping and stacking firewood, gardening and heavy yard work (for example, digging, pushing a wheelbarrow, or laying sod), and chores like shoveling snow also build muscles.

Strength training has gained new respect and has become enormously popular in recent years. Why? Strength training is the single most effective way to increase your amount of lean body mass and to prevent the loss of muscle that occurs as people get older. And, as you add muscle, your metabolic rate increases, causing you to burn more calories and making it easier to lose body fat.

The cosmetic changes that occur with strength training are also very motivating and can be quite dramatic. People soon notice that their body becomes firmer and denser. Their clothes fit looser even if they don't lose weight. This happens because muscle weighs more than fat. For this reason, people should not be discouraged if the number on the scale doesn't drop as quickly as they would like. Let your appearance be your guide, and monitor your results by tracking changes in body measurements or percentage of body fat.

Other benefits of strength training include reduced insulin resistance and lower diabetes risk, since adding muscle enhances the body's ability to remove sugar from the blood. Your bones will become stronger and denser and less likely to fracture. And you will be better able to pursue the activities of daily living, since being stronger staves off the frailty that too often occurs with aging.

How often should you strength train? A total-body strength-training regimen can be accomplished with as little as two one-hour sessions per week. You can strength train in a gym or in the privacy of your own home using an instructional videotape and hand weights. A basic program includes eight to ten different exercises that work the muscles of the legs, trunk, arms, chest and shoulders. However, many people choose to train more intensely and more frequently for larger strength gains and improved muscle tone. Remember, too,

Carbohydrate as Fuel

People who drastically cut carbs from their diet may find they do not have enough energy to engage in high-intensity exercises like weight lifting, sprinting, and fast running. This is because these activities are fueled largely by carbohydrate, which is stored within the muscles as glycogen.

Another important consideration for people engaged in strength-training regimens is that including some carb in your post-workout meal or snack will stimulate muscle building better than a very-low-carb meal will. Why? The insulin released in response to eating some carbohydrate helps shuttle amino acids (the building blocks of protein) into muscles, thereby promoting faster and better gains in lean body mass.

A negative effect on your exercise program is just one more reason to avoid very-low carb ketogenic diet regimens. The Good-Carb Life Plan in Chapter 4 provides a more realistic amount of carbohydrate to support an active lifestyle. People who are very active may need to add even more "good" carbs to their eating plan.

that if you regularly engage in a variety of vigorous activities like gardening, shoveling, and digging, you may not need any additional strength training.

A WORD ABOUT STRETCHING

Remaining flexible is key to maintaining balance and agility throughout life. Being flexible also helps prevent injuries during exercise and everyday activities. You can improve flexibility by stretching at home and/or participating in activities such as yoga, Pilates, and tai chi. Stretch all the major muscle groups at least twice a week, and include stretches as part of your warm-up and cool-down before and after exercise.

IT'S NEVER TOO LATE TO GET STARTED

The great thing about exercise is it's never too late to start. And the older you are, the more you have to gain from being active. Researchers have proven that even people in their nineties can gain strength and perform the activities of daily living much better by adopting an exercise program.

That said, if you have been sedentary for a while, are over age forty-five, are significantly overweight, or are being treated for medical conditions such as heart disease, high blood pressure, prediabetes, or diabetes, you should consult with a physician before embarking on an exercise program. This will give you a chance to have your blood pressure, cholesterol, and blood sugar levels checked. Your doctor may have specific recommendations for exercising based on any physical limitations that you might have.

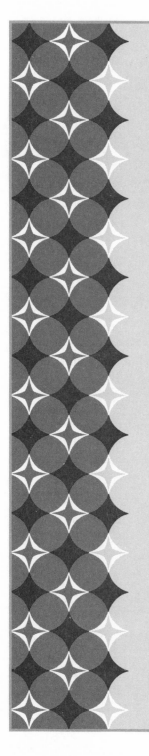

Part II

Recipes for Carb-Conscious Living

About the Recipes and Nutritional Analysis

I'm often amazed at the recipes that are featured in some lower-carb cookbooks. Cups of heavy cream, sticks of butter, gobs of full-fat cheese, and large portions of highly marbled meats, sausages, and bacon. Sound too good to be true? It is. A steady diet like this can pose a serious threat to your future health. Many of these recipes are also astronomically high in calories—but you would have no way of knowing this, since calorie counts are rarely provided.

As I developed these recipes, every effort was made to keep calories under control. Carbs are kept at low to moderate levels, and emphasis is placed on using "good" carbs. Likewise, fats are used moderately with a focus on "good" fats. This allows you to enjoy filling portions of healthful and tasty dishes without blowing your calorie budget or sacrificing your future health.

The Food Processor Nutrition Software (ESHA Research), along with product information from manufacturers, was used to calculate the nutrition information for the recipes in this book. For each recipe, information on calories, carbohydrate, dietary fiber, protein, fat, saturated fat, cholesterol, sodium, and calcium is provided. Nutrients are always given per serving.

Sometimes recipes give options regarding ingredients. For instance, you might be able to choose between eggs or egg substitute, margarine or butter, or nonfat or low-fat milk. This will help you create dishes that suit your tastes and your nutrition goals, but bear in mind that the nutrition analysis is based on the primary ingredient list and does not account for optional ingredients.

8.

Appetizers
and Snacks

No social gathering would be complete without an array of great-tasting finger foods and snacks. But can this be compatible with a lower-carb lifestyle? Absolutely. This chapter will prove that festive occasions need not derail your efforts to eat well. And, with just a little imagination, you can easily whip up an assortment of creative and delicious snacks and never stray from your carb-conscious lifestyle.

Ingredients like low-fat cheeses, lean meats, and light sour cream and mayonnaise can dramatically trim fat and calories from traditional party favorites. "Good" carbs like wholesome whole-grain crackers and whole-wheat tortilla wraps and pitas can also star in your festive fare. This chapter combines these ingredients plus plenty of fresh produce to create a variety of delectable hot and cold hors d'oeuvres that are sure to perk up any party.

Menu-Planning Tips
While on the Low-Carb Quick-Start Plan, limit your choices to items like steamed seafood, lean cold cuts, smoked salmon, lean meatballs in tomato or other nonsweet sauce, low-fat cheeses, and fresh veg-

gies with low-fat dips (like the ones in this chapter), hummus, and tapenade or olivada.

On the Good-Carb Life Plan, you can expand your selections to enjoy any of the above items plus whole-grain crackers and wedges of whole-grain pita bread with light dips and spreads, quesadillas and mini pizzas (like the ones in this chapter), and fresh fruit platters with light yogurt dips.

Mozzarella Bites

Yield: 24 pieces

24 large fresh basil leaves
8 ounce part-skim mozzarella cheese, block or fresh,
 cut into 24 cubes
¼ cup julienned sun-dried tomatoes in olive oil, drained

1. Place the basil leaves with the underside facing up on a platter.
2. Top each leaf with a cube of cheese and ½ teaspoon of the sun-dried toma-toes. Serve immediately.

Nutritional Facts (per piece)
Calories: 29   Carbohydrate: 0.6 g   Cholesterol: 5 mg   Fat: 1.8 g   Saturated Fat: 1 g
Fiber: 0.1 g   Protein: 2.7 g   Sodium: 53 mg   Calcium: 70 mg

Ham & Cheese Skewers

Yield: 12 skewers

3 ounces lean baked ham, cut into 12 (¾-inch) cubes
1 medium scallion, cut into 12 (¾-inch) pieces
12 grape or cherry tomatoes
3 ounces reduced-fat cheddar cheese, cut into 12 (¾-inch) cubes
½ red bell pepper, cut into 12 (¾-inch) pieces
12 large pitted black olives
12 wooden skewers (6-inches each)

1. Thread a ham cube, a scallion piece, a tomato, a cheese cube, a red bell pepper piece, and an olive onto each skewer.
2. Serve immediately, or cover and refrigerate for up to 3 hours before serving.

Nutritional Facts (per skewer)

Calories: 37   Carbohydrate: 2 g   Cholesterol: 6 mg   Fat: 1.6 g   Saturated Fat: 0.6 g   Fiber: 0.4 g   Protein: 4 g   Sodium: 115 mg   Calcium: 66 mg

Light Deviled Eggs

✦ FOR THE MOST NUTRITION, BE SURE TO USE OMEGA-3-
ENRICHED EGGS IN THIS RECIPE.

Yield: 12 pieces

6 hard-boiled eggs
¼ cup nonfat or light mayonnaise
1 tablespoon yellow or spicy brown mustard
2 tablespoons chopped and drained sugar-free sweet pickles
Pinch ground white pepper
Ground paprika

1. Cut the eggs in half lengthwise and remove the yolks. Place the yolks in a small bowl, and mash well. Add the mayonnaise, mustard, pickles, and pepper to the egg yolks, and stir to mix well.
2. Spoon or pipe the yolk mixture into the hollowed-out eggs. Sprinkle some of the paprika over the top of each egg. Transfer to a serving platter and serve immediately, or cover and refrigerate until ready to serve.

Nutritional Facts (per piece)

Calories: 39   Carbohydrate: 1 g   Cholesterol: 95 mg   Fat: 2 g   Saturated Fat: 0.5 g   Fiber: 0 g   Protein: 3 g   Sodium: 102 mg   Calcium: 11 mg

Zucchini-Dill Dip

Yield: about 2 cups

1 cup moderately packed coarsely grated zucchini (about
  1 medium)
½ cup nonfat or light mayonnaise
1 to 2 tablespoons finely chopped fresh dill, or 1 to
  2 teaspoons dried
1 teaspoon fresh or jarred minced garlic
¼ cup finely chopped sweet onion

1. Wrap the zucchini in several layers of cheesecloth or paper towel and squeeze tightly to remove as much of the liquid as possible.
2. Place the zucchini in a medium bowl, add the remaining ingredients, and mix well. Serve immediately or cover and chill until ready to serve. Serve with fresh raw vegetables, sliced smoked salmon, and whole-grain crackers.

Nutritional Facts (per tablespoon)
Calories: 11   Carbohydrate: 2 g   Cholesterol: 1 mg   Fat: 0.1 g   Saturated Fat: 0 g
Fiber: 0.1 g   Protein: 0.5 g   Sodium: 32 mg   Calcium: 13 mg

Sun-Dried Tomato Dip

Yield: about 2¼ cups

1 cup nonfat or light sour cream
1 cup nonfat or light mayonnaise
1½ teaspoons crushed garlic
2 tablespoons finely chopped fresh basil, or 2 teaspoons dried
¼ to ⅓ cup sun-dried tomatoes in olive oil and Italian seasonings
  (drained) plus 1 to 1½ tablespoons of oil from the jar of sun-
  dried tomatoes

1. Combine the sour cream, mayonnaise, garlic, and basil in a medium bowl. Add the oil to the sour cream mixture. Mix well.
2. Chop the tomatoes very finely and stir them into the dip. Cover and chill for

at least 1 hour before serving. Serve with fresh raw vegetables, whole-grain crackers, and rolled-up slices of lean roast beef and turkey.

Nutritional Facts (per tablespoon)

*Calories: 16   Carbohydrate: 2 g   Cholesterol: 0 mg   Fat: 0.3 g   Saturated Fat: 0 g
Fiber: 0.2 g   Protein: 0.5 g   Sodium: 58 mg   Calcium: 11 mg*

Roasted Red Pepper Dip

Yield: about 3 cups

1 cup roasted red pepper, drained and diced
8 ounces reduced-fat (Neufchâtel) cream cheese
¾ cup nonfat or light mayonnaise
1 teaspoon fresh or jarred minced garlic
1 teaspoon dried basil
1 cup shredded Monterey Jack or provolone cheese

1. Place the peppers, cream cheese, mayonnaise, garlic, and basil in a bowl, and beat with an electric mixer to mix well. Beat in the shredded cheese.
2. Serve immediately or chill until ready to serve. Serve with fresh-cut vegetables, rolled-up slices of turkey and lean roast beef, and wedges of whole-grain pita bread.

Nutritional Facts (per tablespoon)

*Calories: 22   Carbohydrate: 0.8 g   Cholesterol: 5 mg   Fat: 1.5 g   Saturated Fat: 0.9 g
Fiber: 0 g   Protein: 1.3 g   Sodium: 60 mg   Calcium: 25 mg*

Carrot-Pecan Cheese Spread

Yield: about 2¼ cups

8 ounces reduced-fat (Neufchâtel) cream cheese
1 to 1½ teaspoons fresh or jarred minced garlic
1½ cups grated carrots (about 3 medium)
¾ cup finely chopped toasted pecans (page 240)
2 tablespoons finely chopped scallions
2 tablespoons finely chopped fresh parsley

1. Place the cream cheese and garlic in a small bowl and beat until smooth. Beat in the carrots, pecans, and scallions.
2. Spread the mixture evenly into a shallow dish and sprinkle the parsley over the top. Serve immediately or cover and chill until ready to serve. Serve with celery sticks, whole-grain crackers, and rolled-up slices of roasted turkey breast.

Nutritional Facts (per tablespoon)

Calories: 36   Carbohydrate: 1 g   Cholesterol: 5 mg   Fat: 3.1 g   Saturated Fat: 1 g   Fiber: 0.4 g   Protein: 1 g   Sodium: 46 mg   Calcium: 8 mg

Spinach-Cheese Spread

Yield: about 3 cups

10-ounce package frozen chopped spinach, thawed and
   squeezed dry
1 8-ounce can water chestnuts, drained and chopped
½ cup thinly sliced scallions
1 cup light vegetable- or garlic-and-herb-flavored cream cheese
½ cup nonfat or light mayonnaise
½ teaspoon dried dill

1. Place the spinach, water chestnuts, and scallions into a medium bowl. Set aside.
2. Place the cream cheese, mayonnaise, and dill in a small bowl and mix well. Add the cream-cheese mixture to the spinach mixture, and mix well. Cover the dip, and chill for at least 1 hour before serving. Serve with fresh-cut vegetables and whole-grain crackers.

Nutritional Facts (per tablespoon)

Calories: 13   Carbohydrate: 1 g   Cholesterol: 3 mg   Fat: 0.7 g   Saturated Fat: 0.4 g   Fiber: 0.4 g   Protein: 0.6 g   Sodium: 41 mg   Calcium: 11 mg

Olive & Sun-Dried Tomato Cheese Log

Yield: 8 servings

8 ounces soft-curd farmer cheese or soft goat cheese

COATING

3 tablespoons chopped sun-dried tomatoes (dry packed)

¼ cup boiling water

⅓ cup chopped black olives

¼ cup (moderately packed) fresh basil

3 tablespoons sliced scallions

1 teaspoon fresh or jarred minced garlic

1. Place the sun-dried tomatoes in a small bowl, and cover with the boiling water. Let sit for 5 minutes, and then drain off the excess liquid.
2. Place the drained tomatoes and all of the remaining coating ingredients in a food processor and process, pulsing the food processor for a few seconds at a time, until the mixture is finely ground. Set aside.
3. Shape the cheese into two 4-inch logs. Spread the olive mixture out on a sheet of waxed paper and roll the cheese logs in the mixture, gently pressing the coating onto the logs to make it stick.
4. Serve immediately or cover and refrigerate until ready to serve. Serve with freshly cut vegetables and whole-grain crackers or wedges of whole-grain pita bread.

Nutritional Facts (per serving)
*Calories: 58   Carbohydrate: 1.6 g   Cholesterol: 9 mg   Fat: 3 g   Saturated Fat: 1.5 g
Fiber: 0.6 g   Protein: 5 g   Sodium: 189 mg   Calcium: 51 mg*

Turkey & Cheese Roll-Ups

Yield: 24 roll-ups

24 slices (4-inch rounds) thinly sliced roasted
    turkey breast (about 12 ounces)

12 slices (4-inch rounds) sliced reduced-fat provolone cheese
(about 6 ounces), cut in half
48 baby arugula or spinach leaves

DRESSING

3 tablespoons nonfat or light mayonnaise
1½ tablespoons Dijon mustard, prepared pesto, or finely chopped
sun-dried tomatoes in olive oil (drained)

1. Place the dressing ingredients in a small bowl and stir to mix.
2. Lay a slice of turkey out on a flat surface. Arrange a half-slice of the cheese over the *bottom half only* of the turkey slice, and spread the cheese with about ½ teaspoon of the dressing. Top the cheese with 2 arugula or spinach leaves, and roll the slice, from the bottom up, to enclose the filling. Repeat with the remaining ingredients to make 24 roll-ups.
3. Secure the roll-ups with a toothpick and serve immediately, or cover and chill until ready to serve.

Nutritional Facts (per roll-up)

Calories: 42   Carbohydrate: 0.5 g   Cholesterol: 14 mg   Fat: 1.6 g   Saturated Fat: 0.1 g   Fiber: 0.1 g   Protein: 6 g   Sodium: 153 mg   Calcium: 63 mg

Artichoke Roll-Ups

Yield: 18 roll-ups

14-ounce can artichoke hearts, well-drained and finely chopped
3 to 4 tablespoons nonfat or light mayonnaise
1½ teaspoons Dijon mustard
18 thin slices (about ½ ounce each) deli roast turkey breast

1. Combine the artichokes, mayonnaise, and mustard in a small bowl and stir to mix well.
2. Lay a slice of turkey out on a flat surface with the short end pointing toward you. Spoon 1 tablespoon of the artichoke mixture along the bottom of the

slice and roll the slice up to enclose the filling. Repeat with the remaining ingredients to make 18 roll-ups.

3. Arrange the roll-ups on a lettuce-lined platter and serve immediately, or cover and refrigerate until ready to serve.

Nutritional Facts (per roll-up)

Calories: 20   Carbohydrate: 2 g   Cholesterol: 5 mg   Fat: 0.1 g   Saturated Fat: 0

Fiber: 0.8 g   Protein: 2.9 g   Sodium: 133 mg   Calcium: 6 mg

Mediterranean Meatballs

Yield: 60 meatballs

MEATBALLS

1¼ pounds 95-percent-lean ground beef

1½ teaspoons fresh or jarred minced garlic

1 teaspoon dried oregano

Scant ½ teaspoon salt

¼ teaspoon ground black pepper

10-ounce package frozen chopped spinach, thawed and
   squeezed dry

1 cup cooked bulgur wheat or brown rice

¾ cup finely chopped onion

SAUCE

2 cups marinara sauce

1. Preheat the oven to 350 degrees. Place all of the meatball ingredients and 2 tablespoons of the marinara sauce in a large bowl, and mix thoroughly.
2. Coat a large baking sheet with nonstick cooking spray. Shape the meatball mixture into 60 1-inch balls, and arrange them in a single layer on the baking sheet. Bake for about 25 minutes, or until nicely browned and no longer pink inside. Transfer the meatballs to a chafing dish or Crock-Pot heated casserole to keep warm.
3. Place the remaining marinara sauce in a small pot, and cook over medium

heat until just heated through. Pour the sauce over the meatballs, toss gently to mix, and serve.

Nutritional Facts (per meatball)

Calories: 20   Carbohydrate: 1.5 g   Cholesterol: 5 mg   Fat: 0.5 g   Saturated Fat: 0.2 g Fiber: 0.3 g   Protein: 2.2 g   Sodium: 52 mg   Calcium: 6 mg

Portobello Pizzas

Yield: 5 servings

5 large portobello mushrooms
4 ounces turkey Italian sausage, casings removed
¼ cup chopped green bell pepper
¼ cup chopped onion
¼ cup plus 1 tablespoon roasted garlic- or Italian-herb-flavored
   tomato paste
1 cup shredded reduced-fat mozzarella cheese

1. Preheat the oven to 450 degrees. Trim the stems from the mushrooms and use a spoon to scrape out the gills, creating a shallow depression in each mushroom. Set aside.
2. Coat a large nonstick skillet with nonstick cooking spray and add the sausage. Cook over medium heat, stirring to crumble, until no longer pink. Drain off and discard any fat. Add the peppers and onions to the skillet, cover, and cook for several minutes, or until the vegetables are tender.
3. Spread 1 tablespoon of the tomato paste in the depression of each mushroom cap, and top the tomato paste in each mushroom with a fifth of the sausage mixture. Place the mushrooms on a baking sheet and bake uncovered for 10 minutes. Top each mushroom with some of the mozzarella cheese and bake for an additional 5 minutes or until the mushrooms are tender and the cheese is lightly browned. Serve hot.

Nutritional Facts (per serving)

Calories: 151   Carbohydrate: 6.5 g   Cholesterol: 50 mg   Fat: 7.3 g   Saturated Fat: 3 g   Fiber: 1.6 g   Protein: 16.5 g   Sodium: 440 mg   Calcium: 211 mg

Spinach and Sun-Dried Tomato Tarts

Yield: 24 pieces

3 to 4 tablespoons sun-dried tomatoes packed in olive oil and
   Italian seasonings (drained), plus 1 tablespoon of oil from the
   jar of sun-dried tomatoes

3 cups (moderately packed) chopped fresh spinach

1 teaspoon fresh or jarred minced garlic

½ teaspoon dried basil

4 pieces whole-wheat or oat-bran pita bread (6-inch rounds)

1 cup shredded reduced-fat mozzarella or provolone cheese

1. Preheat the oven to 400 degrees. Place the oil from the sun-dried tomatoes
   in a medium nonstick skillet. Add the spinach, garlic, and basil. Cook over
   medium-high heat for a couple of minutes or until the spinach wilts. Set aside.

2. Arrange the pitas on a large baking sheet and top each with a quarter of the
   spinach, sun-dried tomatoes, and cheese. Bake for about 8 minutes or until
   the cheese is melted and lightly browned. Cut each tortilla into 6 wedges
   and serve hot.

Nutritional Facts (per piece)

*Calories: 42   Carbohydrate: 5.6 g   Cholesterol: 2 mg   Fat: 1.6 g   Saturated Fat: 0.6 g
Fiber: 0.8 g   Protein: 2.4 g   Sodium: 80 mg   Calcium: 45 mg*

Chicken-Pesto Quesadillas

Yield: 16 pieces

½ cup shredded roasted skinless chicken

2 to 3 teaspoons prepared basil or sun-dried-tomato pesto

½ cup chopped fresh spinach

4 whole-wheat flour tortillas (8-inch rounds)

1 cup shredded reduced-fat mozzarella or provolone cheese

1. Combine the chicken, pesto, and spinach in a small bowl, and toss to mix
   well.

2. Lay a tortilla on a flat surface, and sprinkle the *bottom half only* with 2 table-spoons of the cheese, spreading the cheese to within ½-inch of the edges. Top the cheese with a quarter of the chicken mixture and 2 more table-spoons of cheese. Fold the top half of the tortilla over to enclose the filling. Repeat with the remaining ingredients to make 4 filled tortillas.

3. Coat a large griddle or nonstick skillet with cooking spray, and heat over medium heat until a drop of water sizzles when it hits the heated surface.

4. Lay the quesadillas on the griddle and cook for about 1½ minutes, or until the bottoms are golden brown. Spray the tops lightly with the cooking spray, and then flip with a spatula. Cook for an additional 1½ minutes, or until the second side is golden brown.

5. Transfer the quesadillas to a cutting board, and cut each one into 4 wedges. Serve hot.

Nutritional Facts (per piece)

Calories: 60   Carbohydrate: 6 g   Cholesterol: 8 mg   Fat: 2 g   Saturated Fat: 0.8 g
Fiber: 0.5 g   Protein: 4.5 g   Sodium: 131 mg   Calcium: 36 mg

Turkey-Tapenade Roll-Ups

Yield: 28 pieces

4 whole-wheat flour tortillas (10-inch rounds)
¾ cup light garlic-and-herb-flavored cream cheese spread
8 ounces thinly sliced roasted turkey breast
4 ounces thinly sliced reduced-fat mozzarella cheese
½ cup black olive tapenade or olivada spread
16 very thin slices plum tomato
24 large fresh spinach leaves (about 2 ounces)

1. Spread each tortilla with 3 tablespoons of the cream cheese, extending it all the way to the outer edges. Lay a quarter of the turkey over the *bottom half only* of each tortilla, and top the turkey with a quarter of the cheese, leaving a 1-inch margin on each outer edge. Spread a quarter of the tapenade over the cheese layer, and top with 4 slices of plum tomato. Finish each tortilla off with a layer of spinach leaves.

2. Starting at the bottom, roll each tortilla up tightly. Cut a 1½-inch piece off each end, and discard. Slice the remainder of each tortilla into seven 1-inch pieces. Arrange the rolls on a platter and serve immediately. Or wrap the rolls in plastic wrap, and refrigerate for several hours before slicing and serving.

Nutritional Facts (per piece)

Calories: 55   Carbohydrate: 4.4 g   Cholesterol: 14 mg   Fat: 2.2 g   Saturated Fat: 1.1 g   Fiber: 0.3 g   Protein: 4.5 g   Sodium: 111 mg   Calcium: 40 mg

Pronto Pepperoni Pizzas

Yield: 24 pieces

4 pieces whole-wheat or oat-bran pita bread (6-inch rounds)
1 cup marinara sauce
20 thin slices turkey pepperoni
1 cup shredded reduced-fat mozzarella cheese
3 tablespoons chopped onion
3 tablespoons chopped green bell pepper

1. Arrange the pitas on a large baking sheet and spread some of the marinara sauce over each one.
2. Top each pita with a quarter of the pepperoni, cheese, onions, and bell peppers. Bake at 400 degrees for 8 to 10 minutes, or until the cheese is melted and lightly browned. Cut each pizza into 6 wedges and serve hot.

Nutritional Facts (per piece)

Calories: 43   Carbohydrate: 6 g   Cholesterol: 5 mg   Fat: 1.1 g   Saturated Fat: 0.6 g   Fiber: 0.8 g   Protein: 3 g   Sodium: 135 mg   Calcium: 42 mg

9.

Great Starts—Breakfasts

"Eat to lose" might seem like a paradoxical concept, but this is exactly why breakfast is the most important meal of the day. Eating breakfast and several well-spaced meals throughout the day helps boost your ability to burn calories, maintain more stable blood sugar and insulin levels, and helps ward off overeating later in the day.

Do you skip breakfast because it just makes you feel hungry all day long? Then you may eating the wrong *kind* of breakfast. Breakfast foods like cereal bars, toaster pastries, white bagels, and processed cereals can wreak havoc on your blood sugar, trigger hunger, and cause carbohydrate cravings. Rather than skip breakfast, choose a better breakfast—featuring fiber-rich foods and lean proteins. This chapter offers plenty of ideas that will get your day off to a great start.

Menu-Planning Tips

While on the Quick-Start Plan, limit your choices to items like veggie-filled omelets and other egg dishes, lean breakfast meats, vegetarian sausage or bacon, low-fat cheeses, nonfat or low-fat milk, no-added-sugar yogurt, and low-sodium tomato or vegetable juice.

On the Good-Carb Life Plan, you can expand your selections to enjoy any of the above, plus old-fashioned oatmeal; oat bran; high-fiber, ready-to-eat cereals; whole-grain breads and bran muffins; whole-grain French toast and pancakes (like the recipes in this chapter) topped with a light fruit sauce or light syrup; and assorted fruits.

Mushroom & Herb Omelet

Yield: 1 serving

½ cup sliced fresh mushrooms
½ cup fat-free egg substitute
¼ teaspoon dried chives
⅛ teaspoon dried dill
3 tablespoons shredded reduced-fat Swiss, mozzarella, or white
  cheddar cheese

1. Coat an 8-inch nonstick skillet with cooking spray, and preheat over medium heat. Add the mushrooms, cover, and cook for a couple of minutes, stirring a couple of times, until the mushrooms are tender. Remove the mushrooms to a small dish, and cover to keep warm.
2. Respray the skillet, and return it to the heat. Add the egg substitute and sprinkle the herbs over the top. Reduce the heat to medium-low and cook without stirring for a couple of minutes, or until set around the edges.
3. Use a spatula to lift the edges of the omelet, and allow the uncooked egg to flow below the cooked portion. Cook for another minute or two, or until the eggs are almost set.
4. Arrange first the mushrooms and then the cheese over half of the omelet. Fold the other half over the filling and cook for another minute or two, or until the cheese is melted and the eggs are completely set.
5. Slide the omelet onto a plate, and serve hot.

Nutritional Facts (per serving)
*Calories: 130   Carbohydrate: 3 g   Cholesterol: 11 mg   Fat: 3 g   Saturated Fat: 1.5 g
Fiber: 0.4 g   Protein: 20 g   Sodium: 388 mg   Calcium: 232 mg*

Crab & Chili Omelet

Yield: 1 serving

1 tablespoon canned chopped green chilies
½ cup fat-free egg substitute
¼ cup flaked cooked crabmeat
3 tablespoons shredded reduced-fat Monterey Jack cheese
Ground paprika

1. Coat an 8-inch nonstick skillet with cooking spray, and preheat over medium heat. Stir the chilies into the egg substitute and pour the mixture into the skillet. Reduce the heat to medium-low, then cook without stirring for a couple of minutes, or until set around the edges.
2. Use a spatula to lift the edges of the omelet, and allow the uncooked egg to flow below the cooked portion. Cook for an additional minute or two, or until the eggs are almost set.
3. Arrange first the crabmeat and then the cheese over half of the omelet. Fold the other half over the filling, and cook for another minute or two, or until the cheese is melted and the eggs are completely set.
4. Slide the omelet onto a plate, sprinkle with paprika, and serve hot.

Nutritional Facts (per serving)
Calories: 156   Carbohydrate: 3 g   Cholesterol: 40 mg   Fat: 3.6 g   Saturated Fat: 1.6 g   Fiber: 0.3 g   Protein: 25 g   Sodium: 488 mg   Calcium: 260 mg

Greek Spinach Omelet

Yield: 1 serving

⅓ cup sliced fresh mushrooms
¾ cup (moderately packed) prewashed baby spinach
¼ teaspoon fresh or jarred minced garlic
Pinch ground black pepper
½ cup fat-free egg substitute
1½ tablespoons crumbled reduced-fat feta cheese (plain or with sun-dried tomatoes and herbs)

1 tablespoon chopped seeded plum tomato

⅛ teaspoon dried dill

1. Coat an 8-inch nonstick skillet with cooking spray, and preheat over medium heat. Add mushrooms and cook uncovered for a couple of minutes, stirring frequently, until the mushrooms are tender. Add the spinach, garlic, and pepper, and cook, uncovered, for another minute, or until the spinach is wilted. Remove the mushroom mixture to a small dish, and cover to keep warm.

2. Respray the skillet, and return to the heat. Add the egg substitute, and reduce the heat to medium-low. Cook without stirring for a couple of minutes, or until set around the edges.

3. Use a spatula to lift the edges of the omelet, and allow the uncooked egg to flow below the cooked portion. Cook for another minute or two, or until the eggs are almost set.

4. Arrange first the mushroom mixture and then the cheese over half of the omelet. Fold the other half over the filling and cook for another minute or two, or until the cheese is melted and the eggs are completely set.

5. Slide the omelet onto a plate, top with the tomatoes and dill, and serve hot.

Nutritional Facts (per serving)

Calories: 100   Carbohydrate: 5 g   Cholesterol: 4 mg   Fat: 2 g   Saturated Fat: 1 g

Fiber: 0.8 g   Protein: 16 g   Sodium: 433 mg   Calcium: 114 mg

Chicken Fajita Omelet

Yield: 1 serving

2 tablespoons chopped green bell pepper

2 tablespoons chopped onion

3 tablespoons diced grilled chicken

½ cup fat-free egg substitute

3 tablespoons shredded reduced-fat Monterey Jack or Mexican-
blend cheese

1 tablespoon salsa

1. Coat an 8-inch nonstick skillet with cooking spray, and preheat over medium heat. Add peppers and onion, cover, and cook for a couple of min-

utes, or until tender. Add the chicken and cook for another minute, to heat through. Transfer the mixture to a small dish, and cover to keep warm.

2. Respray the skillet, and return to the heat. Add the egg substitute, and reduce the heat to medium-low. Cook without stirring for a couple of minutes, or until set around the edges.

3. Use a spatula to lift the edges of the omelet, and allow the uncooked egg to flow below the cooked portion. Cook for another minute or two, or until the eggs are almost set.

4. Spread the chicken mixture and 2 tablespoons of the cheese over half of the omelet. Fold the other half over the filling and cook for another minute or two, or until the cheese is melted and the eggs are completely set.

5. Slide the omelet onto a plate, top with the salsa and remaining cheese, and serve hot.

Nutritional Facts (per serving)

Calories: 172   Carbohydrate: 8 g   Cholesterol: 8 mg   Fat: 4.1 g   Saturated Fat: 1.8 g
Fiber: 1.1 g   Protein: 23 g   Sodium: 582 mg   Calcium: 240 mg

Creative Menu Planning

Looking for a change of pace at dinner? Think breakfast. A frittata or omelet served with a bowl of fresh fruit makes for a quick and satisfying meal. By the same token, don't limit yourself to just breakfast foods at breakfast. There's nothing wrong with having some low-fat chicken salad with a wedge of melon, a turkey sandwich on whole-wheat, or even last night's leftovers for breakfast.

Cottage-Style Eggs

Yield: 1 serving

½ cup fat-free egg substitute
2 tablespoons nonfat or low-fat cottage cheese
⅛ teaspoon dried dill

1. Combine the egg substitute, cottage cheese, and dill, and stir to mix. Spray a 2-cup microwave-safe bowl with cooking spray, and add the egg mixture. Microwave at high power for 45 seconds or until the eggs begin to set around the edges and the mixture becomes light and fluffy.
2. Stir the eggs and cook for another minute, or until the eggs are set but not dry. Serve hot.

Nutritional Facts (per serving)

Calories: 80   Carbohydrate: 3 g   Cholesterol: 11 mg   Fat: 0 g   Saturated Fat: 0 g Fiber: 0 g   Protein: 16 g   Sodium: 342 mg   Calcium: 57 mg

Microwave Egg Scramble

Yield: 1 serving

½ cup fat-free egg substitute
2 to 3 tablespoons diced fully cooked lean ham (optional)
3 tablespoons shredded reduced-fat cheddar or Swiss cheese

1. Spray a 2-cup microwave-safe bowl with cooking spray and add the egg substitute and, if desired, the ham. Microwave at high power for 45 seconds or until the eggs begin to set around the edges and the mixture becomes light and fluffy.
2. Stir in the cheese and cook for another minute, or until the eggs are set but not dry. Serve hot.

Nutritional Facts (per serving)

Calories: 126   Carbohydrate: 2 g   Cholesterol: 11 mg   Fat: 3 g   Saturated Fat: 1.5 g Fiber: 0 g   Protein: 19 g   Sodium: 386 mg   Calcium: 248 mg

Zucchini & Sun-Dried Tomato Frittata

Yield: 4 servings

¼ cup julienned or diced sun-dried tomatoes packed in olive oil
(drained), plus 1 tablespoon of oil from the jar of sun-dried
tomatoes

1 medium zucchini, halved lengthwise and sliced

½ teaspoon dried basil

½ teaspoon coarsely ground black pepper

1 teaspoon fresh or jarred minced garlic

2 cups fat-free egg substitute

1 cup shredded reduced-fat mozzarella cheese

1. Preheat the broiler.
2. Spray the bottom and sides of a large nonstick skillet with cooking spray, and add the olive oil from the jar of sun-dried tomatoes. Add the zucchini, basil, and pepper, and sauté over medium-high heat for several minutes, or until the zucchini is crisp-tender. Add the garlic and sun-dried tomatoes, and arrange the mixture evenly over the bottom of the skillet.
3. Pour the egg substitute over the zucchini mixture and reduce the heat to medium-low. Cover and cook without stirring for about 5 minutes or until the edges are set (the top will still be runny).
4. Remove the lid from the skillet and wrap the handle in aluminum foil (to prevent it from becoming damaged under the broiler). Place the skillet under the preheated broiler, and broil for a minute or two, or until the eggs are set but not dry. Sprinkle the cheese over the top and broil for another minute to melt the cheese. Cut the frittata into 4 wedges and serve hot.

Nutritional Facts (per serving)

Calories: 183   Carbohydrate: 6 g   Cholesterol: 16 mg   Fat: 8.9 g   Saturated Fat: 3.4 g   Fiber: 1 g   Protein: 20 g   Sodium: 401 mg   Calcium: 233 mg

Italian Sausage Frittata

Yield: 4 servings

¼ cup grated Parmesan cheese
2 cups fat-free egg substitute
8 ounces turkey Italian sausage, casings removed
1 medium yellow onion, thinly sliced and separated into rings
1 cup (packed) coarsely chopped fresh spinach

1. Preheat the broiler.
2. Stir 2 tablespoons of the Parmesan cheese into the egg substitute. Set aside.
3. Coat the bottom and sides of a large nonstick skillet with cooking spray, and add the sausage. Cook over medium heat, stirring to crumble, until the meat is no longer pink. Add the onion, cover, and cook for a couple of minutes or until the onions are soft. Add the spinach and cook for about 1 minute or until the spinach is just wilted. Arrange the mixture evenly over the bottom of the skillet.
4. Pour the egg substitute over the skillet mixture and reduce the heat to medium-low. Cover and cook without stirring for about 5 minutes or until the eggs are set around the edges (the top will still be runny).
5. Remove the lid from the skillet and wrap the handle in aluminum foil (to prevent it from becoming damaged under the broiler). Place the skillet under the preheated broiler, and broil for a minute or two, or until the eggs are almost set. Sprinkle the remaining Parmesan cheese over the top and broil for another minute or until the eggs are set but not dry. Cut the frittata into 4 wedges and serve hot.

Nutritional Facts (per serving)

Calories: 190   Carbohydrate: 6 g   Cholesterol: 32 mg   Fat: 7.2 g   Saturated Fat: 2.7 g   Fiber: 0.6 g   Protein: 25 g   Sodium: 775 mg   Calcium: 138 mg

Asparagus, Ham, & Egg Bake

Yield: 4 servings

8 ounces thin asparagus spears
Butter-flavored cooking spray

4 ounces thinly sliced, lean, reduced-sodium ham

4 large eggs

3 tablespoons grated Parmesan cheese

1. Preheat the oven to 400 degrees. Rinse the asparagus with cool water and snap off the tough stem ends. Coat 4 small gratin dishes with cooking spray and place a quarter of the asparagus in each dish. Spray the asparagus in each dish lightly with cooking spray and bake uncovered for 7 minutes.

2. Arrange a quarter of the ham over the asparagus in each dish and break an egg over the top of each. Sprinkle a quarter of the Parmesan cheese over each serving. Return the dishes to the oven and bake for an additional 7 minutes or until the egg whites are set and the yolks begin to thicken. Serve hot.

Nutritional Facts (per serving)

Calories: 133   Carbohydrate: 5 g   Cholesterol: 201 mg   Fat: 6.1 g   Saturated Fat: 2 g
Fiber: 0.6 g   Protein: 14 g   Sodium: 411 mg   Calcium: 87 mg

Perfectly Poached Eggs

Poached eggs are a good source of high-quality protein, and the cholesterol contained in an egg a day is not a problem for most people. (Chapter 5 provides more information about the health issues involving eggs.) The easiest way to make poached eggs is to get a microwave egg poacher. This simple cooking device can have your eggs ready in about a minute, with minimal fuss.

To poach eggs the old-fashioned way: Fill a small or medium nonstick skillet (depending on how many eggs you want to poach) with 3 inches of water, and bring to a boil. Reduce the heat to low, to keep the water gently simmering. Break an egg into a custard cup, and, holding the cup at the water's surface, slip the eggs into the water. Repeat for each egg, spacing them evenly apart in the frying pan. Cover and cook for 3 to 5 minutes, or until the whites are completely set and the yolks thickened.

Ham & Eggs Florentine

Yield: 4 servings

4 slices lean reduced-sodium ham (1½ ounces each)

10-ounce package frozen chopped spinach, thawed

4 poached eggs (see the inset "Perfectly Poached Eggs" on
  page 130)

Ground paprika

SAUCE

¼ cup nonfat or light mayonnaise

¼ cup light sour cream

1 tablespoon plus 1 teaspoon Dijon mustard

¼ cup nonfat or low-fat milk

1. Combine all of the sauce ingredients in a microwave-safe bowl and whisk to
   mix well. Set aside.
2. Coat a large nonstick skillet with cooking spray and preheat over medium
   heat. Add the ham and cook for a minute or two on each side or until nicely
   browned. Remove and set aside to keep warm. Add the spinach to the skillet and heat through. Drain off any excess liquid.
3. Place the sauce in a microwave oven, cover, and microwave at 50 percent
   power for about a minute, or until just heated through. Do not let the
   sauce boil.
4. To assemble the dish, place a ham slice on each of 4 serving plates and top
   with a quarter of the spinach, 1 egg, and some of the sauce. Sprinkle some
   paprika over each serving, and serve hot.

Nutritional Facts (per serving)

*Calories: 172   Carbohydrate: 11 g   Cholesterol: 204 mg   Fat: 6.6 g   Saturated Fat: 2 g
Fiber: 2.2 g   Protein: 17 g   Sodium: 669 mg   Calcium: 128 mg*

Eggs Sardou

Yield: 4 servings

SPINACH MIXTURE
4 cups (packed) chopped fresh spinach or 1¼ cups frozen cut
   spinach, thawed
½ cup chopped canned artichoke hearts, well-drained
¼ cup plus 2 tablespoons vegetable- or herb-flavored light
   cream cheese
3 tablespoons nonfat or low-fat milk

4 poached eggs (see "Perfectly Poached Eggs" on page 130)
4 whole-wheat or oat-bran English muffin halves, toasted
Ground paprika

1. To make the spinach mixture, coat a medium nonstick skillet with cooking
   spray, add the spinach, and place over medium heat. Cook for several minutes, stirring frequently, until the spinach is wilted. If using frozen spinach,
   cook only enough to heat through. Then add the artichoke hearts.
2. Add the cream cheese and milk to the spinach mixture. Cook, stirring frequently, until the mixture starts to boil and the cream cheese melts. Add a little more milk if the mixture seems too thick. Set aside and cover to keep warm.
3. To assemble the dish, place one English muffin half on each of 4 serving
   plates. Top each muffin half with a quarter of the spinach mixture and
   1 egg. Sprinkle some paprika over each egg, and serve hot.

Nutritional Facts (per serving)
Calories: 193   Carbohydrate: 19 g   Cholesterol: 205 mg   Fat: 7.8 g   Saturated Fat: 3 g
Fiber: 3.7 g   Protein: 12 g   Sodium: 399 mg   Calcium: 173 mg

Huevos Rancheros

Yield: 1 serving

1 teaspoon extra-virgin olive oil
1 thin corn tortilla (6-inch round)

1 large egg

Ground black pepper

1½ to 2 tablespoons chunky-style salsa

1 tablespoon shredded nonfat or reduced-fat Monterey Jack or
cheddar cheese

¼ cup diced avocado (optional)

1. Place the olive oil in a small nonstick skillet and preheat over medium heat. Add the tortilla, and cook a couple of minutes on each side or until it is lightly browned. Transfer the tortilla to a serving plate.
2. Spray the skillet with cooking spray and crack the egg open into the skillet. Cover and cook over medium-low heat for a minute or two or until the white is mostly set. Flip the egg and cook, covered, for another minute or until the yolk begins to thicken and the white is completely set. Sprinkle the egg lightly with pepper.
3. Place the egg on top of the tortilla and top with the salsa, cheese, and if desired, avocado. Serve hot.

Nutritional Facts (per serving)

Calories: 164   Carbohydrate: 11 g   Cholesterol: 190 mg   Fat: 8.9 g   Saturated Fat: 1.7 g   Fiber: 1.2 g   Protein: 8.5 g   Sodium: 264 mg   Calcium: 98 mg

Sausage & Egg Breakfast Pitas

Yield: 4 servings

6 ounces frozen vegetarian sausage links or patties

¼ cup sliced scallions

1 cup fat-free egg substitute

½ cup shredded reduced-fat Monterey Jack cheese

2 pieces whole-wheat or oat-bran pita bread (6-inch rounds),
cut in half

1. Coat a large nonstick skillet with cooking spray. Add the sausage, cover, and cook over medium heat for several minutes or until the sausage is thawed and beginning to brown. Use a spatula to break the sausage into small pieces. Add the scallions to the skillet, cover, and cook for a couple of

minutes more, or until the sausage is nicely browned and the scallions are tender.

2. Pour the egg substitute over the skillet mixture. Cook over medium-low heat without stirring for a minute or two, or until the eggs are set around the edges. Using a wooden spoon or spatula, begin pushing the eggs to the center of the skillet and stir gently to scramble. Cook until the eggs are just set but not dry. Remove the skillet from the heat, sprinkle the cheese over the top, and let sit for a minute to melt the cheese.

3. Place the pitas on a large plate, cover with a paper towel, and microwave for about 20 seconds to heat through. Fill each pita half with a quarter of the egg mixture and serve hot.

Nutritional Facts (per serving)

Calories: 194   Carbohydrate: 19 g   Cholesterol: 7 mg   Fat: 4.1 g   Saturated Fat: 1.5 g   Fiber: 4 g   Protein: 21 g   Sodium: 688 mg   Calcium: 171 mg

Peach Passion Smoothie

Yield: 1 serving

1 cup frozen (unthawed) sliced peaches, diced
½ cup no-added-sugar vanilla or peach yogurt
½ cup nonfat or low-fat milk
Sugar substitute equal to 1 tablespoon sugar
1–2 tablespoons protein powder (optional)

1. Put all of the ingredients in a blender and blend until smooth.
2. Pour into a tall glass and serve immediately.

Nutritional Facts (per 1½-cup serving)

Calories: 190   Carbohydrate: 36 g   Cholesterol: 5 mg   Fat: 0.4 g   Saturated Fat: 0.2 g   Fiber: 3.4 g   Protein: 11 g   Sodium: 155 mg   Calcium: 359

Triple-Berry Smoothie

Yield: 1 serving

1 cup nonfat or low-fat milk

2 tablespoons nonfat dry milk powder

Sugar substitute equal to 2 tablespoons sugar

½ cup each frozen blueberries, strawberries, and raspberries

1 to 2 tablespoons protein powder (optional)

1. Put all of the ingredients in a blender and blend until smooth.
2. Pour into a tall glass and serve immediately.

Nutritional Facts (per 1½-cup serving)

Calories: 187   Carbohydrate: 35 g   Cholesterol: 5 mg   Fat: 1.5 g   Saturated Fat: 0.3 g   Fiber: 8 g   Protein: 11 g   Sodium: 143 mg   Calcium: 361 mg

Light French Toast

Yield: 10 slices

1 cup fat-free egg substitute

¾ cup evaporated nonfat or low-fat milk

Sugar substitute equal to 1 to 2 tablespoons sugar

¼ teaspoon ground cinnamon

¼ teaspoon vanilla extract

10 slices light or reduced-carbohydrate whole-grain bread

1. Place the egg substitute, evaporated milk, sugar substitute, cinnamon, and vanilla extract in a shallow bowl, and stir with a wire whisk to mix well. Dip the bread slices in the egg mixture, turning to allow both sides to soak up some of the mixture.
2. Coat a large nonstick skillet or griddle with cooking spray, and preheat over medium heat. Lay the bread slices in the skillet and cook for a couple of minutes, or until the bottoms are golden brown. Spray the tops of the bread

slices with the cooking spray, turn, and cook for another minute or two, or until both sides are nicely browned. Serve hot.

Nutritional Facts (per slice)

Calories: 86   Carbohydrate: 9.6 g   Cholesterol: 2 mg   Fat: 1 g   Saturated Fat: 0.2 g   Fiber: 2 g   Protein: 10 g   Sodium: 177 mg   Calcium: 103 mg

French Toast Toppers

Made properly, French toast and even pancakes can fit into your carb-conscious lifestyle. But what do you put on top? After all, just a quarter-cup of pancake syrup contains over 50 grams of carb and 200 calories! Here are some lighter and healthier alternatives.

✦ Fresh berries and a light drizzle of reduced-calorie syrup or honey
✦ Sliced bananas, a light drizzle of reduced-calorie syrup, honey, or maple syrup, and a sprinkling of chopped pecans
✦ Canned no-added-sugar cherry- or apple-pie filling
✦ Fresh fruit sauce like Cherry-Berry Sauce (page 138)
✦ For a quick and easy fruit sauce, purée some canned apricots or peaches, sweeten with a little sugar substitute, and warm in a microwave oven

Ricotta Pancakes

Yield: 20 pancakes

¾ cup whole-wheat pastry flour
Sugar substitute equal to 1 tablespoon sugar
1 teaspoon baking powder
1½ cups nonfat or light ricotta cheese
¾ cup fat-free egg substitute or 3 eggs, lightly beaten
½ cup nonfat or low-fat milk
¾ teaspoon vanilla extract

1. Preheat the oven to 200 degrees.
2. Place the flour, sugar substitute, and baking powder in a medium-sized bowl, and stir to mix well. Combine the ricotta cheese, egg substitute or eggs, milk, and vanilla extract in a small bowl, and stir with a wire whisk to mix well. Add the ricotta mixture to the flour mixture, and whisk until well mixed.
3. Coat a large griddle or nonstick skillet with cooking spray, and preheat over medium heat until a drop of water sizzles when it hits the heated surface. (If using an electric griddle, heat the griddle according to the manufacturer's directions.)
4. For each pancake, pour 3 tablespoons of the batter onto the griddle or skillet and use the back of a spoon to spread the batter into a 3-inch circle. Cook for about 2 minutes, or until the tops are bubbly and the edges are dry. Turn and cook for an additional minute, or until the second side is golden brown. Repeat until all of the batter is used up, respraying the griddle or skillet as necessary.
5. As the pancakes are done, place them on a serving plate, and keep warm in the oven. Serve hot.

Nutritional Facts (per pancake)

Calories: 40   Carbohydrate: 5.5 g   Cholesterol: 1 mg   Fat: 0.1 g   Saturated Fat: 0 g
Fiber: 0.7 g   Protein: 5 g   Sodium: 64 mg   Calcium: 114 mg

Blueberry–Buttermilk Pancakes

Yield: 16 pancakes

¾ cup oat bran
¾ cup whole-wheat pastry flour
Sugar substitute equal to 2 tablespoons sugar
1 teaspoon baking powder
½ teaspoon baking soda
1¾ cups nonfat or low-fat buttermilk
¼ cup fat-free egg substitute
1½ cups fresh or frozen (unthawed) blueberries

1. Preheat the oven to 200 degrees.
2. Place the oat bran, flour, sugar substitute, baking powder, and baking soda

in a medium bowl, and stir to mix well. Add the buttermilk and egg substitute to the flour mixture, and whisk to mix well. Fold in the blueberries.

3. Coat a large griddle or nonstick skillet with cooking spray, and preheat over medium heat until a drop of water sizzles when it hits the heated surface. (If using an electric griddle, heat the griddle according to manufacturer's directions.)

4. For each pancake, pour ¼ cup of the batter onto the griddle or skillet and use the back of a spoon to spread the batter into a 4-inch circle. Cook for about 1½ minutes, or until the tops are bubbly and the edges are dry. Turn and cook for an additional minute, or until the second side is golden brown. Repeat until all of the batter is used up, respraying the griddle or skillet as necessary.

5. As the pancakes are done, place them on a serving plate, and keep warm in the oven. Serve hot.

Nutritional Facts (per pancake)

Calories: 52   Carbohydrate: 11 g   Cholesterol: 1 mg   Fat: 0.7 g   Saturated Fat: 0.2 g Fiber: 2 g   Protein: 3 g   Sodium: 107 mg   Calcium: 53 mg

Cherry-Berry Sauce

◆ THIS FLAVORFUL SAUCE HAS JUST A FRACTION OF THE CARBS OF PANCAKE SYRUP AND IS LOADED WITH ESSENTIAL NUTRIENTS.

Yield: about 1½ cups

¼ cup white grape juice
1½ teaspoons cornstarch
1½ cups fresh or frozen pitted sweet cherries, coarsely chopped
1½ cups fresh or frozen blueberries
Sugar substitute equal to 2½ tablespoons sugar

1. Place 1 tablespoon of grape juice and all the cornstarch in a small bowl. Stir to dissolve the cornstarch, and set aside.

2. Place the cherries and blueberries, the remaining juice, and the sugar substitute in a 1½-quart saucepan. Cover, and cook over medium heat, stirring

occasionally for about 5 minutes, or until the fruit begins to break down and release its juices.

3. Stir the cornstarch mixture, and add it to the pot. Cook, stirring constantly, for another minute or two, or until the mixture is thickened and bubbly. Serve hot.

Nutritional Facts (per ¼-cup serving)
Calories: 56   Carbohydrate: 13 g   Cholesterol: 0 mg   Fat: 0.2 g   Saturated Fat: 0 mg   Fiber: 2 g   Protein: 0.5 g   Sodium: 1 mg   Calcium: 10 mg

Molasses Bran Muffins

Yield: 12 muffins

1 cup bran-flake-and-raisin cereal
1 cup nonfat or low-fat milk
¼ cup plus 2 tablespoons fat-free egg substitute
¼ cup molasses
2 tablespoons canola oil
1½ cups oat bran
¼ cup brown sugar
2 teaspoons baking powder
½ cup chopped walnuts
⅓ cup chopped dried apricots or raisins

1. Preheat oven to 375 degrees.
2. Place the cereal, milk, egg, molasses, and oil in a bowl and stir to mix. Set aside for at least 10 minutes.
3. Combine the oat bran, brown sugar, and baking powder in a medium bowl and stir to mix well. Press out any lumps in the brown sugar. Add the cereal mixture to the oat-bran mixture and stir to mix. Stir in the walnuts and the apricots or raisins.
4. Coat the bottoms only of muffin cups with cooking spray, and divide the batter among the muffin cups. Bake at 375 degrees for about 15 minutes, or until a wooden toothpick inserted in the center of a muffin comes out clean.

5. Remove the muffin tin from the oven, and allow it to sit for 5 minutes before removing the muffins. Serve warm or at room temperature.

Nutritional Facts (per 1 muffin)

Calories: 154   Carbohydrate: 24 g   Cholesterol: 0 mg   Fat: 6.2 g   Saturated Fat: 0.6 g   Fiber: 3 g   Protein: 5 g   Sodium: 98 mg   Calcium: 56 mg

Oatmeal Breakfast Bread

Yield: 16 slices

1 cup whole-wheat pastry flour
⅔ cup old-fashioned (5-minute) or quick-cooking (1 minute) oats
2 teaspoons baking powder
½ teaspoon baking soda
⅓ cup light-brown sugar
1 cup nonfat or low-fat buttermilk
3 tablespoons canola oil
¼ cup fat-free egg substitute
1 teaspoon vanilla extract
⅓ cup chopped walnuts or toasted pecans (page 240)
⅓ cup chopped dried apricots, dried cherries or blueberries,
   or raisins

1. Preheat the oven to 350 degrees.
2. Place the flour, oats, baking powder, and baking soda in a medium bowl, and stir to mix well. Add the brown sugar and stir to mix. Use the back of a spoon to press out any lumps in the brown sugar.
3. Add the buttermilk, oil, egg substitute, and vanilla, and stir to mix well. Set the batter aside for 10 minutes. Add the nuts and fruit and stir to mix well.
4. Coat an 8-by-4-inch pan with cooking spray and spread the batter evenly in the pan. Bake for about 40 minutes or until a wooden toothpick inserted in the center of the loaf comes out clean. Let the bread cool in the pan for 15 minutes, then invert onto a wire rack to cool to room temperature.

Nutritional Facts (per slice)

Calories: 111   Carbohydrate: 15 g   Cholesterol: 0 mg   Fat: 4.8 g   Saturated Fat: 0.5 g   Fiber: 2 g   Protein: 2.7 g   Sodium: 126 mg   Calcium: 61 mg

10.

Savory Soups
and Stews

Made with light and healthy ingredients, soups and stews can be a real boon to the carb-conscious menu planner. A steaming cup of vegetable soup is the perfect partner to a main dish salad or hearty sandwich, while a savory bowl of chili or beef stew makes a satisfying hot and hearty entrée. And even when you take the time to make soup from scratch, you'll find that soups and stews are perfect for a busy lifestyle. Most can be prepared ahead of time, and then refrigerated or frozen until needed. In fact, soups and stews usually taste even better when refrigerated overnight, allowing the flavors to marry and blend.

The recipes in this chapter feature lean meats, poultry, legumes, and whole grains combined with plenty of garden vegetables and savory seasonings. The result is a selection of soups and stews that are bursting with flavor, brimming with important nutrients, and just right for your lower-carb lifestyle.

Menu-Planning Tips

While on the Quick-Start Plan, choose soups and stews made with lean proteins, legumes, low-fat milk and cheese, and plenty of low-carb vegetables.

On the Good-Carb Life Plan you can expand your selection to enjoy soups and stews made with moderate portions of whole-wheat pastas and whole grains like brown rice, wild rice, and barley.

Sicilian Vegetable Beef Soup

Yield: 11 servings

1 pound 95-percent-lean ground beef
1 medium yellow onion, chopped
½ cup chopped celery
1 cup diced carrot
4½ cups water
14½-ounce can diced tomatoes with roasted garlic or
   Italian seasonings
1½ cups vegetable juice cocktail
1 tablespoon beef bouillon granules
¼ teaspoon ground black pepper
1 teaspoon dried Italian seasoning
15-ounce can white beans, drained
1 cup whole-wheat macaroni, uncooked
2 cups (packed) fresh spinach, sliced

1. Coat a 4-quart pot with cooking spray and add the ground beef. Cook over medium heat, stirring to crumble, until the meat is no longer pink. Add the onions and celery, cover, and cook for several minutes more, or until the vegetables start to soften.
2. Add the carrots, water, undrained tomatoes, vegetable juice, bouillon granules, pepper, and Italian seasoning to the pot, and bring to a boil. Reduce the heat, cover, and simmer for 20 minutes.
3. Add the beans and macaroni, and cook covered for about 6 minutes or until the macaroni is almost al dente. Add the spinach, and cook for another minute or two, or until the spinach is wilted. Serve hot.

Nutritional Facts (per 1-cup serving)
Calories: 123   Carbohydrate: 16 g   Cholesterol: 22 mg   Fat: 2.1 g   Saturated Fat: 0.8 g   Fiber: 3.2 g   Protein: 12 g   Sodium: 480 mg   Calcium: 53 mg

Beef & Barley Soup

Yield: 11 servings

1 pound 95-percent-lean ground beef

1 medium-large yellow onion, chopped

½ cup chopped celery

4 cups sliced fresh mushrooms

1 cup diced carrot

6 cups water

14½-ounce can diced tomatoes with roasted garlic or
   Italian seasonings

½ cup pearl barley

1½ tablespoons dried parsley

1½ tablespoons beef bouillon granules

1 teaspoon dried thyme

¼ teaspoon ground black pepper

1 cup frozen green peas

1. Coat a 4-quart pot with cooking spray and add the ground beef. Cook over medium heat, stirring to crumble, until the meat is no longer pink. Add the onions, celery, and mushrooms, cover, and cook for several minutes more, or until the vegetables start to soften.

2. Add the carrots, water, undrained tomatoes, barley, parsley, bouillon granules, thyme, and pepper to the pot, and bring to a boil. Reduce the heat, cover, and simmer for 45 minutes.

3. Add the peas and cook covered for an additional 15 minutes, or until the barley and peas are tender. Serve hot.

Nutritional Facts (per 1-cup serving)

Calories: 123   Carbohydrate: 15 g   Cholesterol: 22 mg   Fat: 2.1 g   Saturated Fat: 0.8 g   Fiber: 3.1 g   Protein: 11 g   Sodium: 459 mg   Calcium: 33 mg

Burgundy Beef Stew

Yield: 6 servings

1½ pounds lean stew beef, cut in bite-sized pieces

1 tablespoon extra-virgin olive oil

6 cups fresh mushrooms, halved (about 1 pound)

2 teaspoons dried thyme

1½ teaspoons fresh or jarred minced garlic

1 teaspoon ground paprika

1 teaspoon coarsely ground black pepper

1½ cups dry red wine

2 teaspoons beef bouillon granules

1½ cups and 1 tablespoon water

2 cups frozen pearl onions

1 tablespoon cornstarch

1. Rinse the meat and pat dry with paper towels. Coat a large nonstick skillet with cooking spray and preheat over medium-high heat. Brown the meat in 2 batches and transfer to a 4-quart nonstick pot. Set aside.

2. Add the olive oil and mushrooms to the skillet. Cook for several minutes, or until nicely browned. Add the thyme, garlic, paprika, and pepper to the skillet, and stir to mix. Transfer the mixture to the pot containing the beef, along with the wine and bouillon granules.

3. Pour 1½ cups of the water into the skillet and use a spatula to scrape up the browned bits from the bottom. Pour the mixture into the pot containing the beef. Bring the pot to a boil, then reduce the heat to low. Cover and simmer for 1 hour and 45 minutes or until the beef is fork tender. Add the onions and bring to a boil. Reduce the heat and simmer, covered, for 10 minutes more, or until the onions are tender.

4. Dissolve the cornstarch into 1 tablespoon of water and pour into the pot. Cook and stir for a couple of minutes or until the sauce thickens. Serve hot.

Nutritional Facts (per 1-cup serving)

Calories: 263   Carbohydrate: 9 g   Cholesterol: 84 mg   Fat: 9 g   Saturated Fat: 3.2 g
Fiber: 1.4 g   Protein: 24 g   Sodium: 269 mg   Calcium: 29 mg

Chipotle Black Bean Chili

Yield: 8 servings

1 pound 95-percent-lean ground beef or turkey

1 cup chopped onion

14½-ounce can diced tomatoes with roasted garlic, undrained

8-ounce can unsalted tomato sauce

2 tablespoons chili powder

3 to 4 teaspoons finely chopped canned chipotle chilies in
    adobo sauce★

1 teaspoon ground cumin

¾ teaspoon dried oregano

2 15-ounce cans black beans, undrained

Toppings (optional)

¾ cup shredded nonfat or reduced-fat Monterey Jack or
    cheddar cheese

½ cup sliced scallions or chopped red onions

1. Coat a 3-quart pot with cooking spray and add the ground beef. Place over medium heat and cook, stirring to crumble, until the meat is no longer pink. Drain off and discard any fat. Add the onions, cover, and cook for several minutes, or until the onions are tender.
2. Add the remaining ingredients except for the beans, and bring to a boil. Reduce the heat to low, cover, and simmer for 15 minutes.
3. Add the beans and simmer for 10 minutes more. Serve hot, topping each serving with some cheese and scallions or onions if desired.

Nutritional Facts (per 1-cup serving)

Calories: 193   Carbohydrate: 21 g   Cholesterol: 30 mg   Fat: 3.9 g   Saturated Fat: 1.1 g   Fiber: 7.7 g   Protein: 18 g   Sodium: 478 mg   Calcium: 61 mg

---

★ Chipotle chiles in abodo sauce are smoked red jalapeño peppers that are canned in a tomato-vinegar sauce. Small cans can be found in the Mexican section of most grocery stores. Leftovers can be frozen in ice-cube trays and transferred to freezer bags for later use. Be sure to wear gloves when working with all hot peppers as the hot components can cause a burning sensation.

Lentil Soup with Italian Sausage

Yield: 7 servings

8 ounces mild Italian sausage, casings removed, sliced ¼-inch thick★

1 cup chopped onion

¾ cup chopped celery

¾ cup chopped carrot

5 cups water

1½ cups lentils

1 teaspoon chicken or vegetable bouillon granules

2 teaspoons fresh or jarred minced garlic

¾ teaspoon dried Italian seasoning

1. Coat a 4-quart pot with cooking spray and add the sausage. Cook over medium heat for several minutes or until the sausage is nicely browned.
2. Add the remaining ingredients to the pot and bring the mixture to a boil. Reduce the heat to low, cover, and cook for about 1 hour or until the lentils are soft and the liquid is thick. Serve hot.

Nutritional Facts (per 1-cup serving)
Calories: 195   Carbohydrate: 26 g   Cholesterol: 27 mg   Fat: 3.5 g   Saturated Fat: 1 g Fiber: 9.5 g   Protein: 16 g   Sodium: 523 mg   Calcium: 33 mg

★ Partially freezing the sausage will make it easier to slice.

Spinach & White Bean Soup

Yield: 7 servings

1 tablespoon extra-virgin olive oil

1 cup chopped onion

4 cups reduced-sodium chicken broth

1 teaspoon dried Italian seasoning

1 cup diced lean, reduced-sodium ham

2 teaspoons fresh or jarred minced garlic

15-ounce can white beans, drained

½ cup whole-wheat macaroni or other small pasta, uncooked

4 cups chopped fresh spinach

1. Place the olive oil in a 2½-quart nonstick pot and place over medium heat. Add the onions, cover, and cook for several minutes or until the onions start to soften. Add the broth, Italian seasoning, ham, and garlic, and bring to a boil. Reduce the heat to low, cover, and simmer for 10 minutes.

2. Mash about ¼ cup of the white beans and add to the pot along with the remaining beans. Add the pasta to the pot and bring to a boil. Reduce the heat to medium-low, cover, and cook for about 8 minutes or until the pasta is almost al dente. Add the spinach and cook for another minute or two, or until the spinach is wilted and the pasta is al dente. Serve hot, topping each serving with a sprinkling of grated Parmesan cheese if desired.

Nutritional Facts (per 1-cup serving)

Calories: 198   Carbohydrate: 28 g   Cholesterol: 16 mg   Fat: 3 g   Saturated Fat: 0.5 g   Fiber: 4.3 g   Protein: 15 g   Sodium: 420 mg   Calcium: 70 mg

Split Pea Soup with Bacon

Yield: 5 servings

1 medium yellow onion, chopped

½ cup diced carrot

1 teaspoon fresh or jarred minced garlic

4 cups chicken broth

1¼ cups dried green split peas

2 bay leaves

1 teaspoon dried rosemary

Scant ¼ teaspoon ground black pepper

2 to 3 slices turkey bacon, cooked and crumbled

1. Coat a 2½-quart nonstick pot with cooking spray and place over medium heat. Add the onions, cover, and cook for several minutes or until the onions soften. Add the remaining ingredients except for the bacon, and bring to a boil.

2. Reduce the heat to low and simmer, covered, for about 1 hour. Serve hot, topping each serving with some of the bacon.

Nutritional Facts (per 1-cup serving)

Calories: 169   Carbohydrate: 29 g   Cholesterol: 4 mg   Fat: 1 g   Saturated Fat: 0.2 g Fiber: 11 g   Protein: 12 g   Sodium: 475 mg   Calcium: 25 mg

Zesty Gazpacho

Yield: 5 servings

1¾ cups vegetable juice cocktail
½ cup picante sauce or salsa
3 tablespoons red wine vinegar
1½ tablespoons extra-virgin olive oil
2 teaspoons sugar substitute or sugar
1½ teaspoons fresh or jarred minced garlic
1 teaspoon chili powder
2 cups diced tomatoes (about 2 large)
1½ cups diced, peeled, and seeded cucumber (about 1½ medium)
½ cup diced green bell pepper
½ cup diced yellow or orange bell pepper
½ cup chopped Spanish or sweet onion
½ cup light sour cream (optional)

1. Place the vegetable juice, picante sauce or salsa, vinegar, olive oil, sugar substitute or sugar, garlic, and chili powder in a medium-size bowl, and stir to mix well.
2. Place tomatoes, cucumbers, bell peppers, and onions in the bowl of a food processor, and pour the vegetable juice mixture over the vegetables. Process the mixture for several seconds, or until the vegetables are finely chopped.
3. Transfer the soup to a covered container and chill for 2 to 6 hours. Serve chilled, topping each serving with a dollop of sour cream if desired.

Nutritional Facts (per 1-cup serving)

Calories: 94   Carbohydrate: 13 g   Cholesterol: 0 mg   Fat: 4.5 g   Saturated Fat: 0.6 g Fiber: 3 g   Protein: 2 g   Sodium: 357 mg   Calcium: 25 mg

Summer Squash Soup

Very Good

Yield: 4 servings

1 tablespoon margarine or butter

½ cup chopped onion

1 large yellow bell pepper, chopped

5 cups sliced yellow squash

1½ teaspoons fresh or jarred minced garlic

1½ cups chicken broth

Scant ½ teaspoon salt

⅛ teaspoon ground black pepper

2 tablespoons finely chopped fresh parsley or dill, or 2 teaspoons
   dried parsley or dill, finely crumbled

1. Place the margarine or butter in a 2-quart pot and place over medium heat. Add the onions and bell pepper, cover, and cook for several minutes, or until the onions and pepper are softened. Add the squash, garlic, broth, salt, and ground black pepper, and bring to a boil. Reduce the heat to low, cover, and simmer for about 10 minutes or until the squash is soft.

2. Transfer the soup, half at a time, to a blender, and carefully blend at low speed until smooth. Return the puréed soup to the pot and reheat for a minute or two. Add a little more broth if needed. Serve hot, topping each serving with a sprinkling of the parsley or dill.

Nutritional Facts (per 1-cup serving)

Calories: 70   Carbohydrate: 11 g   Cholesterol: 0 mg   Fat: 2.7 g   Saturated Fat: 0.7 g
Fiber: 4 g   Protein: 2.4 g   Sodium: 470 mg   Calcium: 40 mg

Italian Vegetable Soup

Yield: 7 servings

1 tablespoon extra-virgin olive oil

1 medium yellow onion, cut into thin wedges

3 cups water

14½-ounce can diced tomatoes with Italian seasonings, puréed in
a blender until smooth
1½ cups small cauliflower florets
¾ cup diced carrot
1 teaspoon fresh or jarred minced garlic
1 teaspoon Italian seasoning
¼ teaspoon salt
¼ teaspoon ground black pepper
1½ cups small broccoli florets
1½ cups sliced yellow or zucchini squash

1. Place the olive oil in a 3-quart nonstick pot and add the onions. Cover and
   cook over medium heat for several minutes or until the onions begin to
   soften. Add the water, tomatoes, cauliflower, carrots, garlic, Italian seasoning, salt, and pepper. Bring the mixture to a boil, then reduce the heat to
   low. Cover, and simmer for 10 minutes.
2. Add the broccoli florets to the soup, cover, and simmer for 5 minutes. Add
   the squash, cover, and simmer for an additional 5 minutes or until the vegetables are tender. Serve hot.

Nutritional Facts (per 1-cup serving)
*Calories: 62   Carbohydrate: 8 g   Cholesterol: 0 mg   Fat: 2.1 g   Saturated Fat: 0.3 g
Fiber: 2.9 g   Protein: 2.5 g   Sodium: 247 mg   Calcium: 44 mg*

Savory Butternut Squash Soup

Yield: 5 servings

2 medium butternut squash (¾ pound each), halved lengthwise
and seeded
1½ tablespoons extra-virgin olive oil
1 cup chopped onion
1 teaspoon dried sage
⅛ teaspoon ground black pepper
3 cups chicken or vegetable broth
⅓ cup shredded Parmesan cheese

1. Preheat oven to 400 degrees. Coat a large baking sheet with cooking spray and lay the squash halves, cut-side down, on the sheets. Bake for about 45 minutes, or until soft. Let the squash cool and scoop out the flesh. (There should be about 2 cups of squash.)

2. Place the olive oil in a 2½-quart pot and add the onions. Cover and cook over medium heat for about 4 minutes, stirring several times, or until the onions are soft.

3. Place the sautéed onions, sage, pepper, broth, and squash in a blender and blend until smooth. Pour the blended soup back into the pot and bring to a boil. Reduce the heat to low, cover, and simmer for 5 minutes. Serve hot, topping each serving with some of the Parmesan cheese.

Nutritional Facts (per 1-cup serving)

Calories: 109   Carbohydrate: 12 g   Cholesterol: 5 mg   Fat: 5.6 g   Saturated Fat: 1.6 g   Fiber: 2.9 g   Protein: 4.1 g   Sodium: 468 mg   Calcium: 120 mg

Cauliflower-Cheese Soup

Yield: 5 servings

1 tablespoon margarine or butter
1 medium-small yellow onion, chopped
1 teaspoon dried savory
6 cups fresh cauliflower florets
1½ cups chicken broth
⅛ teaspoon ground white pepper
2 cups nonfat or low-fat milk
3 ounces processed reduced-fat cheddar cheese (like Lifetime or Velveeta Light), diced
3 tablespoons thinly sliced scallions, or 2 slices turkey bacon, cooked and crumbled

1. Add the margarine or butter to a 2½-quart nonstick pot and melt over medium heat. Add the onions and savory, cover, and cook for several minutes or until the onions soften (do not let them brown).

2. Add the cauliflower, broth, and pepper, and bring to a boil. Reduce the heat to medium-low and simmer for 10 minutes or until the cauliflower is tender.

3. Pour the soup mixture and about half of the milk into a blender and carefully blend at low speed with the lid slightly ajar (to allow steam to escape) until the mixture is smooth. Return the mixture to the pot and add the remaining milk.

4. Place the blended soup over medium heat and cook, stirring frequently, until heated through. Stir in the cheese and cook for another minute or two to melt the cheese. Serve hot, topping each serving with a sprinkling of the scallions or bacon.

Nutritional Facts (per 1-cup serving)

Calories: 129   Carbohydrate: 15 g   Cholesterol: 9 mg   Fat: 4 g   Saturated Fat: 1.8 g Fiber: 3.5 g   Protein: 9.4 g   Sodium: 568 mg   Calcium: 251 mg

11.

Light and Easy Entrées

Many people believe that adopting a carb-conscious lifestyle means spending hours in the kitchen preparing complicated recipes and purchasing an array of special, exorbitantly priced low-carb ingredients. As you will see, nothing could be further from the truth. This chapter will prove that healthful and delicious meals can be easily prepared using ingredients that are widely available in your local grocery store.

Menu-Planning Tips

While on the Quick-Start Plan, limit your main-dish choices to lean meats, seafood, skinless poultry, and vegetarian alternatives like tofu, veggie burgers, and legumes.

On the Good-Carb Life Plan you can expand your selections to enjoy any of the above, plus moderate portions of whole-grain pasta and dishes containing whole grains like brown rice, wild rice, and barley. And when planning your lower-carb meals, be sure to balance your entrée with the appropriate side dishes. For instance, if you are having a pasta entrée like Roasted Red Pepper Lasagna, pair it with a fresh garden salad and a low-carbohydrate vegetable like green beans or asparagus. Add other starches like a piece of crusty whole-grain bread only if you need the extra carbohydrates and calories.

Balsamic Chicken

◆ FOR VARIETY, SUBSTITUTE PORK TENDERLOIN FOR THE CHICKEN.

Yield: 4 servings

½ teaspoon dried rosemary
½ teaspoon dried sage
¼ teaspoon garlic powder
¼ teaspoon ground black pepper
¼ teaspoon salt
1 pound boneless skinless chicken breast, cut into 8 equal pieces
    and pounded ½-inch thick
1 tablespoon extra-virgin olive oil
¼ cup balsamic vinegar
¼ cup chicken broth
2 tablespoons finely chopped fresh parsley or 2 teaspoons dried
    parsley, finely crumbled

1. Combine the rosemary, sage, garlic powder, pepper, and salt, and sprinkle some of the mixture over both sides of the chicken pieces.
2. Coat a large nonstick skillet with the olive oil, and preheat over medium-high heat. Add the chicken and cook for a couple of minutes on each side or until nicely browned. Cover the skillet and reduce the heat to medium. Cook for about 3 minutes, turning once, until the chicken is thoroughly cooked. Remove the chicken from the skillet and set aside to keep warm.
3. Add the vinegar and broth to the skillet, and cook and stir over medium-high heat for several minutes or until reduced to about 3 tablespoons in volume.
4. To serve, divide the chicken among 4 serving plates, drizzle with some of the sauce, and top with a sprinkling of parsley. Serve hot.

Nutritional Facts (per serving)

Calories: 167   Carbohydrate: 2.7 g   Cholesterol: 66 mg   Fat: 4.9 g   Saturated fat:
0.9 g   Fiber: 0.2 g   Protein: 26 g   Sodium: 292 mg   Calcium: 12 mg

Sicilian Stuffed Chicken Breasts

Yield: 4 servings

½ cup chopped canned artichoke hearts, drained

3 tablespoons sun-dried tomatoes packed in olive oil, drained

2 tablespoons grated Parmesan cheese or crumbled blue cheese

½ teaspoon dried basil

4 boneless skinless chicken breast halves (5 ounces each)

½ teaspoon salt

½ teaspoon ground black pepper

1 tablespoon extra-virgin olive oil

1. Combine the artichoke hearts, tomatoes, cheese, and basil in a small bowl, and toss to mix well. Set aside.
2. Cut a deep pocket into the thickest side of each piece of chicken and stuff a quarter of the artichoke mixture into each pocket. Close by pressing flesh together and secure with a wooden toothpick if necessary. Sprinkle both sides of the chicken pieces with some of the salt and pepper.
3. Pour the olive oil into a large nonstick skillet and preheat over medium-high heat. Add the chicken and cook for a couple of minutes on each side or until nicely browned. Reduce the heat to medium-low, cover, and cook for about 8 to 10 minutes, turning occasionally, until the chicken is cooked through. Serve hot.

Nutritional Facts (per serving)

Calories: 220   Carbohydrate: 3.5 g   Cholesterol: 84 mg   Fat: 6.8 g   Saturated fat:
1.6 g   Fiber: 1.5 g   Protein: 35 g   Sodium: 468 mg   Calcium: 69 mg

Bistro Chicken

Yield: 4 servings

2 pounds bone-in skinless chicken breast, legs, or thighs

½ teaspoon garlic powder

½ teaspoon coarsely ground black pepper

1 tablespoon extra-virgin olive oil

1 medium onion, chopped

½ cup chopped celery

¼ cup plus 2 tablespoons white zinfandel wine or chicken broth

1 teaspoon dried basil

1 to 2 tablespoons capers

1 teaspoon dried parsley, finely crumbled, or 3 tablespoons finely
  chopped fresh parsley

14½-ounce can diced tomatoes with Italian seasonings

1. Sprinkle both sides of the chicken with some of the garlic powder and pepper. Coat a large nonstick skillet with the olive oil and preheat over medium–high heat. Add the chicken and cook for a couple of minutes on each side, or until nicely browned.

2. Spread the onions and celery around the chicken pieces and reduce the heat to medium. Cover and cook for about 5 minutes, stirring occasionally, until the vegetables are tender. Pour the wine or broth into the skillet, cover, and cook for another couple of minutes.

3. Add the capers, basil, half of the parsley, and the undrained tomatoes to the skillet and bring to a boil. Reduce the heat to low, cover, and simmer for about 25 minutes or until the chicken is very tender and no longer pink inside. Simmer uncovered for a few minutes if the sauce seems too thin. Sprinkle the remaining parsley over the top and serve hot. Serve with whole-wheat couscous or pasta if desired.

Nutritional Facts (per serving, white meat)

Calories: 283   Carbohydrate: 9 g   Cholesterol: 98 mg   Fat: 5.5 g   Saturated fat: 1.1 g   Fiber: 2.3 g   Protein: 41 g   Sodium: 442 mg   Calcium: 71 mg

Nutritional Facts (per serving, dark meat)

Calories: 300   Carbohydrate: 9 g   Cholesterol: 136 mg   Fat: 9.9 g   Saturated fat: 2.1 g   Fiber: 2.3 g   Protein: 36 g   Sodium: 478 mg   Calcium: 71 mg

Chicken Athenos

Yield: 4 servings

1 pound chicken breast tenders, or 1 pound boneless skinless
    chicken breast, cut into 8 pieces and pounded ½-inch thick
1 tablespoon Greek Spice Rub (page 76) or Greek seasoning
1 tablespoon extra-virgin olive oil
2 cups sliced fresh mushrooms
1 medium yellow onion, chopped
¼ cup plus 2 tablespoons chopped sun-dried tomatoes (dry pack)
½ cup white zinfandel wine
1 cup coarsely chopped canned artichoke hearts, drained
¼ cup crumbled reduced-fat feta cheese

1. Rub some of the spice mixture over both sides of each piece of chicken. Coat a large nonstick skillet with the olive oil and preheat over medium-high heat. Add the chicken and cook for a couple of minutes on each side, or until nicely browned.
2. Remove the chicken from the skillet and set aside. Add the mushrooms and onions to the skillet, cover, and cook over medium heat for several minutes or until tender.
3. Add the chicken back to the skillet. Scatter the sun-dried tomatoes around the chicken and pour the wine over the top. Cover and cook over medium-low heat for 10 minutes.
4. Transfer 2 pieces of chicken to each of 4 serving plates. Add the artichoke hearts to the skillet mixture and cook over medium-high for a minute to heat through. Spoon one quarter of the vegetable mixture and pan juices over each piece of chicken. Top each serving with a tablespoon of the feta cheese and serve hot.

Nutritional Facts (per serving)
Calories: 275   Carbohydrate: 12 g   Cholesterol: 85 mg   Fat: 6.5 g   Saturated fat: 1.6 g   Fiber: 4.2 g   Protein: 37 g   Sodium: 413 mg   Calcium: 76 mg

Quick Chicken Cacciatore

Yield: 4 servings

1 pound chicken breast tenders, or 1 pound boneless skinless
    chicken breast, cut into 8 pieces and pounded ½-inch thick
½ teaspoon coarsely ground black pepper
½ teaspoon garlic powder
1 medium yellow onion, sliced and separated into rings
1 cup sliced fresh mushrooms
1 tablespoon extra-virgin olive oil
14½-ounce can diced tomatoes with Italian seasonings
2 tablespoons roasted garlic-flavor tomato paste
¼ cup grated Parmesan cheese
2 cups cooked whole-wheat angel-hair pasta (optional)

1. Sprinkle some of the pepper and garlic powder over both sides of each piece of chicken and set aside.
2. Coat a large nonstick skillet with cooking spray and place over medium-high heat. Add the onions and mushrooms, cover, and cook for several minutes, stirring occasionally, until the vegetables are tender. Remove the vegetables from the skillet and set aside.
3. Add the olive oil to the skillet, and preheat over medium-high heat. Add the chicken and cook for a couple of minutes on each side or until nicely browned. Place the sautéed vegetables over the chicken and pour the tomatoes over the top. Cover and cook for about 10 minutes or until the chicken is thoroughly cooked and tender. Stir the tomato paste into the pan juices. Serve hot (over ½ cup of pasta if desired), topping each serving with a tablespoon of the Parmesan cheese.

Nutritional Facts (per serving)
Calories: 244   Carbohydrate: 14 g   Cholesterol: 70 mg   Fat: 6.8 g   Saturated fat: 2 g
Fiber: 2 g   Protein: 31 g   Sodium: 652 mg   Calcium: 160 mg

Cider-Glazed Chicken

Yield: 4 servings

1 pound chicken breast tenders, or 1 pound boneless skinless
   chicken breast, cut into 8 pieces and pounded ½-inch thick
¾ teaspoon dried rosemary
½ teaspoon garlic powder
½ teaspoon coarsely ground black pepper
½ teaspoon salt
1 tablespoon canola oil

GLAZE

½ cup apple cider or apple juice
¼ cup low-sodium chicken broth
1 teaspoon Dijon mustard
2 tablespoons finely chopped fresh parsley, or 2 teaspoons dried
   parsley, finely crumbled

1. Rinse the chicken and pat dry with paper towels. Combine the rosemary, garlic powder, pepper, and salt, and rub some of the mixture over both sides of the chicken.
2. Place the canola oil in a large nonstick skillet and preheat over medium-high heat. Add the chicken tenders and cook for a couple of minutes on each side, or until nicely browned. Reduce the heat to medium-low, cover, and cook for about 3 minutes more, or until the chicken is cooked through. Remove the chicken from the skillet and set aside to keep warm.
3. Add the apple juice, broth, and mustard to the skillet and cook over medium-high heat for several minutes or until the mixture is reduced to about ¼ cup in volume. To serve, place a quarter of the chicken tenders on each of 4 serving plates and drizzle each with some of the glaze. Top each serving with some of the parsley. Serve hot.

Nutritional Facts (per serving)

*Calories: 172   Carbohydrate: 4 g   Cholesterol: 66 mg   Fat: 5 g   Saturated fat: 0.7 g
Fiber: 0.2 g   Protein: 26 g   Sodium: 397 mg   Calcium: 20 mg*

Chicken Tenders with Spicy Black Beans

Yield: 4 servings

1 pound chicken breast tenders

1 teaspoon ground cumin

½ teaspoon garlic powder

½ teaspoon coarsely ground black pepper

¼ teaspoon salt

1 tablespoon extra-virgin olive oil

1 cup canned black beans, undrained

½ cup chunky-style salsa

½ cup shredded reduced-fat Monterey Jack or Mexican-blend
   cheese (optional)

3 tablespoons finely chopped fresh cilantro or thinly sliced
   scallions

1. Rinse the chicken and pat dry with paper towels. Combine the cumin, garlic powder, pepper, and salt, and rub some of the mixture over both sides of the chicken tenders.

2. Place the olive oil in a large nonstick skillet and preheat over medium-high heat. Add the chicken tenders and cook for a couple of minutes on each side, or until nicely browned. Reduce the heat to medium, cover, and cook for about 3 minutes more or until the chicken is cooked through. Remove the chicken from the skillet and set aside to keep warm.

3. Add the black beans and salsa to the skillet and cook over medium-high heat for a minute or two to heat through. To serve, place a quarter of the chicken tenders on each of 4 serving plates and top with a quarter of the black-bean mixture. If desired, top each serving with some of the cheese and sprinkle with some of the cilantro or scallions. Serve hot.

Nutritional Facts (per serving)
Calories: 201   Carbohydrate: 14 g   Cholesterol: 66 mg   Fat: 4.9 g   Saturated fat:
0.8 g   Fiber: 3.5 g   Protein: 29 g   Sodium: 629 mg   Calcium: 37 mg

Lemon Chicken

Yield: 4 servings

SAUCE

¼ cup dry sherry

¼ cup chicken broth

1 tablespoon lemon juice

2 tablespoons small capers

1 pound boneless skinless chicken breast

2 teaspoons lemon pepper

3 tablespoons whole-wheat pastry flour, or unbleached flour

1 tablespoon extra-virgin olive oil

3 tablespoons finely chopped fresh parsley

1. Stir together the sauce ingredients and set aside.
2. Rinse the chicken with cool water, pat it dry with paper towels, and cut into 8 equal pieces. Pound each piece to ¼-inch thickness and sprinkle some of the lemon pepper over both sides of the chicken pieces. Dredge the chicken in the flour, turning to coat all sides.
3. Pour the olive oil into a large nonstick skillet, and preheat over medium-high heat. Add the chicken and cook for 2 to 3 minutes on each side or until nicely browned and no longer pink inside. Remove the chicken from the skillet and set aside to keep warm.
4. Add the sauce to the skillet, and cook for a couple of minutes, stirring frequently, until the mixture is reduced by about half and thickens slightly.
5. To serve, place 2 chicken pieces on each of 4 serving plates and top with some of the sauce and a sprinkling of parsley. Serve hot.

Nutritional Facts (per serving)

Calories: 187   Carbohydrate: 5 g   Cholesterol: 65 mg   Fat: 4.8 g   Saturated Fat: 0.8 g   Fiber: 0.3 g   Protein: 27 g   Sodium: 365 mg   Calcium: 17 mg

Tequila-Lime Chicken

Yield: 4 servings

SAUCE
¼ cup orange juice
2 tablespoons lime juice
2 tablespoons tequila
1 tablespoon honey

1 pound boneless skinless chicken breast
½ teaspoon ground cumin
½ teaspoon dried oregano
½ teaspoon salt
¼ teaspoon garlic powder
¼ teaspoon ground black pepper
1 tablespoon extra-virgin olive oil
¼ cup finely chopped fresh cilantro, or thinly sliced scallions

1. Stir together the sauce ingredients and set aside.
2. Rinse the chicken with cool water, pat it dry with paper towels, and cut into 8 equal pieces. Pound each piece to ¼-inch thickness. Stir together the cumin, oregano, salt, garlic powder, and pepper, and sprinkle some of the mixture over both sides of the chicken pieces.
3. Pour the olive oil into a large nonstick skillet and preheat over medium-high heat. Add the chicken and cook for 2 to 3 minutes on each side or until nicely browned and no longer pink inside. Remove the chicken from the skillet and set aside to keep warm.
4. Add the sauce to the skillet, and cook for a couple of minutes, stirring frequently, until the mixture is reduced by about half and thickens slightly.
5. To serve, place 2 chicken pieces on each of 4 serving plates and top with some of the sauce and a sprinkling of cilantro or scallions. Serve hot.

Nutritional Facts (per serving)

Calories: 196   Carbohydrate: 7 g   Cholesterol: 66 mg   Fat: 4.8 g   Saturated Fat: 0.8 g
Fiber: 0.8 g   Protein: 26 g   Sodium: 365 mg   Calcium: 16 mg

Mushroom Meatloaf

Yield: 8 servings

1½ pounds 95-percent-lean ground beef or ground turkey

2 cups very finely chopped fresh mushrooms

¾ cup very finely chopped onion

¾ cup quick-cooking (1-minute) oats

8-ounce can tomato sauce with roasted garlic or Italian herbs

¼ cup plus 2 tablespoons fat-free egg substitute

¼ cup very finely chopped fresh parsley, or 1 tablespoon plus
   1 teaspoon dried parsley

½ teaspoon coarsely ground black pepper

½ teaspoon salt

1. Place all of the ingredients except for ½ cup of the tomato sauce in a large bowl, and mix well. Coat a 9-by-5-inch meatloaf pan with nonstick cooking spray and press the mixture into the pan to form a loaf.
2. Bake uncovered at 350 degrees for 35 minutes. Spread the remaining tomato sauce over the meatloaf and bake for 30 additional minutes, or until the meat is no longer pink inside and a meat thermometer reads at least 160 degrees.
3. Remove the loaf from the oven, and let sit for 10 minutes before slicing and serving.

Nutritional Facts (per serving)

Calories: 160   Carbohydrate: 9 g   Cholesterol: 45 mg   Fat: 4.4 g   Saturated Fat: 1.6 g   Fiber: 1.7 g   Protein: 20 g   Sodium: 399 mg   Calcium: 18 mg

Cube Steak with Mushrooms, Peppers, & Onions

Yield: 4 servings

½ teaspoon garlic powder

¼ teaspoon ground black pepper

½ teaspoon salt

1 pound beef cube steak, cut into 4 equal pieces

2 cups sliced fresh mushrooms

1 green bell pepper, cut into thin strips

1½ medium yellow onions, sliced and separated into rings

1. Coat a large nonstick skillet with cooking spray and preheat over medium-high heat. Combine the garlic powder, pepper, and half of the salt, and sprinkle some over both sides of the steak pieces. Cook the steaks for a couple of minutes on each side, or until nicely browned.

2. Spread the mushrooms, peppers, and onions over the steaks. Cover the skillet and reduce the heat to medium-low. Cook the steaks for about 10 minutes, turning once, or until the steaks and vegetables are tender. Add a little water or broth during cooking if the skillet becomes too dry, but only enough to prevent scorching.

3. Remove the steaks from the skillet and set aside to keep warm. Sprinkle the remaining salt over the vegetables and toss to mix. If necessary, cook the vegetable mixture over medium-high heat for a minute or two, or until any excess liquid evaporates and the vegetables are nicely browned. Serve hot, topping each serving with some of the vegetables.

Nutritional Facts (per serving)

Calories: 203   Carbohydrate: 7 g   Cholesterol: 76 mg   Fat: 4.5 g   Saturated Fat: 1.5 g   Fiber: 2 g   Protein: 33 g   Sodium: 332 mg   Calcium: 17 mg

Moussaka

Yield: 6 servings

1-pound eggplant, cut into ½-inch thick rounds

½ teaspoon coarsely ground black pepper

FILLING

1 pound 95-percent-lean ground beef or turkey

1 medium yellow onion, chopped

1 teaspoon fresh or jarred minced garlic

½ teaspoon dried basil

½ teaspoon dried oregano

¼ teaspoon ground allspice or cinnamon

8-ounce can roasted garlic or Italian herb-flavored tomato sauce

3 tablespoons roasted garlic or Italian herb-flavored tomato paste

SAUCE

3 tablespoons unbleached flour

2 cups nonfat or low-fat milk

¼ cup plus 2 tablespoons fat-free egg substitute

⅛ teaspoon salt

¼ cup plus 2 tablespoons grated Parmesan cheese

1. Preheat the oven to 450 degrees.
2. Coat a large baking sheet with cooking spray and arrange the eggplant slices on the sheet. Sprinkle with the pepper and spray the tops lightly with cooking spray. Bake 10 minutes. Turn the slices and bake for an additional 6 minutes or until tender and golden brown. Set aside, and reduce the oven temperature to 350 degrees.
3. To make the filling, coat a large nonstick skillet with cooking spray and add the ground meat. Place over medium heat and cook, stirring to crumble, until the meat is no longer pink. Drain off and discard any fat. Add the onion, garlic, basil, oregano, and allspice or cinnamon. Cover and cook for several minutes more or until the onion is tender. Add the tomato sauce and paste. Cover and simmer for 5 minutes. Keep covered and set aside to keep warm.
4. To make the sauce, place the flour in a 2-quart glass bowl, add about ¼ cup of the milk, and whisk until smooth. Slowly whisk in the remaining milk and then the egg substitute and salt. Microwave at high power for 2 minutes, then whisk until smooth. (The mixture may appear curdled at first but will become smooth as you keep whisking.) Microwave for about 3 minutes more, whisking after each minute, until thickened and bubbly.
5. To assemble the casserole, coat an 8-inch square baking dish with cooking spray and arrange half of the eggplant slices over the bottom of the dish. Sprinkle 2 tablespoons of the Parmesan cheese over the eggplant slices and top with all of the ground-meat filling. Cover the filling with the remaining eggplant slices, 2 tablespoons of Parmesan, and all of the sauce. Sprinkle the remaining Parmesan over the top and spray the top lightly with cooking spray.

6. Bake uncovered for about 30 minutes or until the edges are bubbly. Remove the dish from the oven and let sit for 20 minutes before serving. To serve, cut into squares, and carefully lift each piece out with a spatula. Serve hot.

Nutritional Facts (per serving)
Calories: 217   Carbohydrate: 17 g   Cholesterol: 47 mg   Fat: 5.6 g   Saturated Fat: 2.7 g   Fiber: 3.1 g   Protein: 24 g   Sodium: 525 mg   Calcium: 205 mg

Spaghetti Squash Casserole

Yield: 6 servings

2½-pound spaghetti squash
2 tablespoons water
1 pound 95-percent-lean ground beef or turkey
1 medium yellow onion, chopped
2 cups chopped fresh mushrooms
1 teaspoon fresh or jarred minced garlic
14½-ounce can diced tomatoes with Italian seasonings
½ teaspoon dried sage or oregano
¼ teaspoon ground black pepper
3 tablespoons grated Parmesan cheese
1 cup shredded reduced-fat mozzarella cheese

1. Preheat oven to 350 degrees.
2. Cut the squash in half lengthwise and remove the seeds. Place the squash halves cut-side down in a 9-by-13-inch microwave safe dish and add the water. Cover loosely with microwave-safe plastic wrap. Microwave at high power for about 12 to 15 minutes or until the squash is easily pierced with a fork. Set the squash aside to cool, then scoop out the pulp and separate it into strands with a fork. (This step can be done the day before to save time.)
3. Coat a large nonstick skillet with cooking spray and add the ground meat. Cook, stirring to crumble, until the meat is no longer pink. Add the onions, mushrooms, and garlic, cover, and cook for several minutes or until the vegetables are tender. Add the tomatoes, sage or oregano, and pepper, and cook uncovered for several minutes, or until most of the liquid has evaporated.

4. Add the squash to the meat mixture and toss gently to mix. Coat a 9-by-13-inch pan with cooking spray and spread the mixture evenly in the dish. Sprinkle the Parmesan over the top, and bake uncovered at 350 degrees for 25 minutes or until heated through. Top with the mozzarella and bake for another 5 minutes to melt the cheese. Let sit for 10 minutes before serving.

Nutritional Facts (per serving)
Calories: 223   Carbohydrate: 16 g   Cholesterol: 53 mg   Fat: 7.2 g   Saturated Fat: 3.4 g   Fiber: 3.8 g   Protein: 24 g   Sodium: 394 mg   Calcium: 170 mg

Zucchini Lasagna

Yield: 6 servings

1 pound zucchini (about 3 medium), cut lengthwise into
   ½-inch thick slices
½ teaspoon coarsely ground black pepper

MEAT FILLING
1 pound 95-percent-lean ground beef, or turkey Italian sausage,
   casings removed
1 medium yellow onion, chopped
¾ teaspoon dried Italian seasoning (omit if using Italian sausage)
14½-ounce can diced tomatoes with Italian seasonings
3 tablespoons roasted garlic– or Italian herb–flavored tomato paste

RICOTTA FILLING
¾ cup nonfat or reduced-fat ricotta cheese
1½ tablespoons fat-free egg substitute

¼ cup grated Parmesan cheese
1 cup shredded reduced-fat mozzarella cheese

1. Preheat oven to 450 degrees.
2. Coat a large baking sheet with cooking spray and arrange the zucchini slices on the sheet. Sprinkle with the pepper and spray the tops lightly with cook-

ing spray. Bake for 10 minutes. Turn the slices over and bake for an additional 5 minutes or until tender and nicely browned. Set aside, and reduce the oven temperature to 350 degrees.

3. To make the meat filling, coat a large nonstick skillet with cooking spray and add the ground beef or sausage. Place over medium heat and cook, stirring to crumble, until the meat is no longer pink. Drain off and discard any fat. Add the onions and Italian seasoning. Cover and cook for several minutes more or until the onions are tender. Add the undrained tomatoes and tomato paste. Simmer uncovered for a couple of minutes or until the mixture is thick. Set aside.

4. To make the ricotta filling, combine the ricotta and egg substitute in a small bowl and stir to mix well. Set aside.

5. To assemble the casserole, coat an 8-inch square baking dish with cooking spray and arrange half of the zucchini slices over the bottom of the dish. Sprinkle 2 tablespoons of the Parmesan cheese over the zucchini slices and top with half of the meat filling. Dot all of the ricotta filling over the meat filling. Layer on the remaining zucchini, Parmesan, and meat filling.

6. Bake uncovered for 20 minutes. Sprinkle the mozzarella cheese over the top and bake for an additional 10 minutes or until the edges are bubbly and the cheese is melted. Remove the dish from the oven and let sit for 20 minutes before serving. To serve, cut into squares, and carefully lift each piece out with a spatula. Serve hot.

Nutritional Facts (per serving)

Calories: 213   Carbohydrate: 12 g   Cholesterol: 50 mg   Fat: 6 g   Saturated Fat: 2.8 g
Fiber: 2.3 g   Protein: 26.5 g   Sodium: 458 mg   Calcium: 278 mg

Balsamic Braised Beef Roast

Yield: 7 servings

3-pound well-trimmed lean pot roast such as top round, eye
   round, or bottom round
½ teaspoon coarsely ground black pepper
½ teaspoon garlic powder
¼ teaspoon salt
2 cups beef broth

½ cup balsamic vinegar

1 teaspoon dried thyme

1 teaspoon dried rosemary

1. Rinse the meat with cool water and pat it dry with paper towels. Sprinkle the pepper, garlic powder, and salt over all sides of the meat.
2. Coat a nonstick 6-quart pot or Dutch oven with cooking spray and preheat over medium-high heat. Place the meat in the pot or Dutch oven and cook for several minutes, or until all sides are nicely browned.
3. Add the broth, balsamic vinegar, thyme, and rosemary to the pot, and let the mixture come to a boil. Reduce the heat to low, cover, and simmer for about 2½ hours, turning the roast occasionally, until fork tender. Remove the roast to a cutting board, cover loosely with foil, and let sit for 10 minutes.
4. Strain the pan juices through a wire strainer into a fat separator cup. Return the defatted juices back to the pot and boil uncovered over medium-high heat until reduced to 1¼ cups in volume. Slice the meat very thinly across the grain and serve hot with the pan juices.
5. *Slow Cooker Method:* Brown the meat as directed and place in a 3-quart or larger slow cooker. Reduce the broth to 1 cup and cook the roast at high power for about 4 hours or low power for 8 to 10 hours or until fork tender.

Nutritional Facts (per 3-ounce serving)

Calories: 180   Carbohydrate: 3 g   Cholesterol: 73 mg   Fat: 4.7 g   Saturated Fat: 1.6 g   Fiber: 0 g   Protein: 29 g   Sodium: 291 mg   Calcium: 8 mg

Savory Slow-Cooked Brisket

Yield: about 8 servings

3-pound well-trimmed flat half beef brisket or top round roast

1¼ teaspoons coarsely ground black pepper

¾ teaspoon salt

1 large Spanish onion, chopped (about 3 cups)

2 to 3 teaspoons fresh or jarred minced garlic

1¼ teaspoons ground paprika

1¼ cups beef broth

1. Rinse the roast and pat it dry with paper towels. Sprinkle both sides with the salt and pepper. Coat a large nonstick skillet with cooking spray and preheat over medium-high heat. Add the brisket and cook for several minutes on each side or until nicely browned. Transfer to a 3-quart or larger slow cooker.

2. Respray the skillet and add the onions and a couple of tablespoons of water. Cover and cook over medium heat for about 5 minutes, stirring occasionally until the onions soften. Stir in the garlic and paprika and cook for another 30 seconds. Add the broth and bring the mixture to a boil.

3. Pour the onion mixture over and around the brisket. Cover and cook at high power for 5 hours or at low power for 10 hours or until the brisket is very tender.

4. Remove the brisket to a cutting board and cover loosely with foil. Set aside to keep warm.

5. Strain the pan juices into a fat separator cup, then pour the defatted juices into a 1½-quart pot. Boil over medium-high heat for several minutes or until the juices are reduced to about 1 cup in volume. Serve the brisket hot accompanied by the pan juices.

Nutritional Facts (per 3-ounce cooked, trimmed serving)
Calories: 181   Carbohydrate: 2 g   Cholesterol: 80 mg   Fat: 5.4 g   Saturated Fat: 1.8 g   Fiber: 0.3 g   Protein: 27 g   Sodium: 373 mg   Calcium: 18 mg

Herb-Roasted Pork Loin

Yield: 8 servings

2 pounds well-trimmed boneless pork loin roast
2 to 3 tablespoons Greek, Caribbean, or Cajun Spice Rub (page 76) or your favorite herb seasoning blend
Olive oil cooking spray

1. Preheat oven to 350 degrees.
2. Rinse the roast and pat it dry with paper towels. Rub the seasoning over all sides of the roast.
3. Coat a 9-by-13-inch pan with the cooking spray and lay the roast in the pan. Spray the top of the roast with the cooking spray.
4. Bake uncovered for 50 to 60 minutes, or until a meat thermometer reads

155 to 160 degrees for medium or 165 to 170 degrees for well-done. Cover the roast loosely with aluminum foil and let sit for 15 minutes before thinly slicing and serving.

Nutritional Facts (per 3-ounce serving)
*Calories: 154   Carbohydrate: 1 g   Cholesterol: 74 mg   Fat: 7 g   Saturated Fat: 2.6 g
Fiber: 0.2 g   Protein: 21 g   Sodium: 230 mg   Calcium: 20 mg*

Savory Stuffed Pork Chops

Yield: 4 servings

2 slices multigrain or oatmeal bread
1 cup chopped fresh mushrooms
½ cup finely chopped onions
⅓ cup finely chopped celery (include some leaves)
½ teaspoon poultry seasoning
½ teaspoon salt
4 well-trimmed 1-inch-thick boneless pork loin chops (about
    5 ounces each)
¼ teaspoon ground black pepper
1 tablespoon extra-virgin olive oil

1. Tear the bread into chunks, place in a food processor, and process into coarse crumbs. Set aside.
2. Coat a large nonstick skillet with cooking spray. Add the mushrooms, onions, celery, poultry seasoning, and half of the salt. Cover and cook over medium-high heat for about 4 minutes, stirring several times, until the vegetables are tender. Add a little water or broth if the skillet becomes too dry. Remove from the heat and toss in the bread crumbs. Add a tablespoon of water if necessary to moisten the crumbs enough to make the mixture hold together.
3. Cut a deep pocket into the thickest side of each pork chop and stuff a quarter of the mushroom mixture into each pocket. Close by pressing flesh together and secure with a wooden toothpick if necessary. Sprinkle both sides of the pork chops with some of the remaining salt and the pepper.
4. Wipe out the skillet, add the olive oil, and preheat over medium-high heat. Add the pork chops and cook for a couple of minutes on each side or until

nicely browned. Reduce the heat to medium-low, cover, and cook for about 8 to 10 minutes, turning occasionally, until the pork chops are cooked through. Serve hot.

Nutritional Facts (per serving)

Calories: 252   Carbohydrate: 10 g   Cholesterol: 82 mg   Fat: 7.8 g   Saturated fat: 1.7 g   Fiber: 1.7 g   Protein: 35 g   Sodium: 434 mg   Calcium: 9 mg

Peppercorn Pork Chops

Yield: 4 servings

4 well-trimmed boneless pork center loin chops (4 ounces each)
2 teaspoons cracked black peppercorns
¼ teaspoon salt
1 tablespoon olive or canola oil

SAUCE
¼ cup dry sherry
¼ cup chicken broth
2 teaspoons Dijon mustard

1. Rinse the pork chops with cool water and pat dry with paper towels. Rub some of the peppercorns and salt over both sides of the chops.
2. Place the oil in a large nonstick skillet and preheat over medium-high heat. Add the pork chops and cook for a couple of minutes on each side, or until nicely browned. Reduce the heat to medium-low, cover, and cook for about 8 minutes, turning the chops occasionally, until they are cooked through. Remove the chops from the skillet and set aside.
3. To make the sauce, add the sherry, broth, and mustard to the skillet and increase the heat to medium-high. Cook uncovered, whisking frequently, for several minutes or until the mixture is reduced by half and thickens slightly. Drizzle the sauce over the pork chops and serve hot.

Nutritional Facts (per serving)

Calories: 176   Carbohydrate: 1 g   Cholesterol: 67 mg   Fat: 6.7 g   Saturated fat: 1.5 g   Fiber: 0.2 g   Protein: 26 g   Sodium: 351 mg   Calcium: 27 mg

Raspberry Pork Medallions

Yield: 4 servings

SAUCE
¼ cup plus 2 tablespoons chicken broth
¼ cup light (low-sugar) raspberry fruit spread
1 tablespoon white wine vinegar or balsamic vinegar
1½ teaspoons Dijon mustard

1 pound pork tenderloin
1 teaspoon dried rosemary or thyme
¼ teaspoon garlic powder
¼ teaspoon salt
¼ teaspoon coarsely ground black pepper
1 tablespoon canola oil
3 tablespoons thinly sliced scallions

1. Place all of the sauce ingredients in a bowl and stir to mix well. Set aside.
2. Rinse the tenderloin with cool water, pat dry with paper towels, and cut crosswise into 8 equal pieces. Use the palm of your hand or a meat mallet to flatten each piece to ½-inch thickness. Combine the rosemary or thyme, garlic powder, salt, and pepper, and sprinkle some of the mixture over both sides of each pork medallion. Set aside.
3. Place the oil in a large nonstick skillet and preheat over medium-high heat. Add the pork medallions and cook for a couple of minutes on each side or until nicely browned and no longer pink inside. Remove the medallions from the skillet and set aside to keep warm.
4. Pour the sauce into the skillet and cook, stirring frequently, for a couple of minutes, or until sauce is reduced by almost half and is syrupy.
5. To serve, place 2 pieces of pork on each of 4 serving plates. Drizzle each serving with some of the sauce and top with a sprinkling of scallions. Serve hot.

Nutritional Facts (per serving)
Calories: 177   Carbohydrate: 7 g   Cholesterol: 76 mg   Fat: 6.1 g   Saturated fat: 1.3 g   Fiber: 0.3 g   Protein: 24 g   Sodium: 302 mg   Calcium: 13 mg

Grilled Rosemary Pork

Yield: 4 servings

1 pound pork tenderloin
1½ teaspoons Dijon or spicy mustard
½ teaspoon garlic powder
½ teaspoon coarsely ground black pepper
¼ teaspoon salt
1 tablespoon extra-virgin olive oil
10 to 12 sprigs (4 to 6 inches each) fresh rosemary

1. Rinse the tenderloin and pat dry with paper towels. Stir together the mustard, garlic powder, pepper, salt, and half of the olive oil, and spread over the tenderloin, coating all sides.
2. Cover the tenderloin on all sides with the rosemary sprigs, and tie in several places with kitchen twine to secure the rosemary to the tenderloin. Drizzle the remaining olive oil over the rosemary.
3. Place the tenderloin on a grill rack and grill, covered, over medium coals for about 20 minutes, turning occasionally, until a thermometer inserted in the thickest part of the meat reads 155 to 160 degrees. Remove the tenderloin from the grill, cover loosely with foil, and let sit for 5 minutes before slicing thinly at an angle. Serve immediately.

Nutritional Facts (per serving)
*Calories: 164   Carbohydrate: 2 g   Cholesterol: 67 mg   Fat: 6 g   Saturated Fat: 1.7 g
Fiber: 0.7 g   Protein: 24 g   Sodium: 241 mg   Calcium: 20 mg*

Cajun Shrimp

Yield: 4 servings

1¼ pounds peeled and de-veined large shrimp
3 to 4 teaspoons Cajun Spice Rub (page 76) or Cajun seasoning
1 tablespoon plus 1 teaspoon extra-virgin olive oil

1. Rinse the shrimp with cool water and pat dry with paper towels. Place the shrimp in a large bowl, sprinkle with the Cajun seasoning, and toss to mix.

2. Coat a large nonstick skillet with the olive oil and preheat over medium-high heat. Add the shrimp and cook, stirring frequently for several minutes, until the shrimp turn pink and are cooked through. Serve hot.

Nutritional Facts (per serving)

Calories: 195   Carbohydrate: 2 g   Cholesterol: 215 mg   Fat: 7 g   Saturated Fat: 1 g   Fiber: 0.2 g   Protein: 29 g   Sodium: 382 mg   Calcium: 85 mg

Grilled Southwestern Shrimp with Mango Salsa

Yield: 4 servings

1½ pounds large shrimp
1 tablespoon plus 1 teaspoon Southwestern seasoning*
1 tablespoon extra-virgin olive oil

MANGO SALSA
1½ cups diced fresh mango
¼ cup plus 2 tablespoons finely chopped red onion
¼ cup finely chopped fresh cilantro
¼ cup finely chopped green bell pepper
1 teaspoon lime juice
⅛ teaspoon salt

1. Peel and de-vein the shrimp, leaving the tails on. Toss with the Southwestern seasoning and olive oil, and set aside.
2. Combine all of the salsa ingredients in a bowl, and toss to mix. Set aside.
3. Thread a quarter of the shrimp onto each of four 12-inch skewers. Grill over medium coals for about 3 minutes on each side or until the shrimp turn opaque. Serve hot, accompanied by the salsa.

Nutritional Facts (per serving)

Calories: 246   Carbohydrate: 15 g   Cholesterol: 232 mg   Fat: 6.5 g   Saturated Fat: 1 g   Fiber: 2.1 g   Protein: 32 g   Sodium: 487 mg   Calcium: 99 mg

---

* Combine 1½ teaspoons chili powder, 1 teaspoon ground cumin, ½ teaspoon paprika, ½ teaspoon salt, ¼ teaspoon coarsely ground black pepper, and ¼ teaspoon garlic powder, or use a ready-made Southwestern seasoning.

Pan-Seared Scallops

Yield: 4 servings

3 tablespoons whole-wheat pastry flour
½ teaspoon dried thyme
½ teaspoon ground paprika
Scant ½ teaspoon salt
¼ teaspoon ground black pepper
1¼ pounds large scallops, rinsed and patted dry
1 tablespoon plus 1 teaspoon extra virgin olive oil or canola oil
Olive-oil or butter-flavored cooking spray
Lemon wedges

1. Place the flour, thyme, paprika, salt, and pepper in a shallow dish and mix well. Add the scallops and toss to coat. Set aside.
2. Coat a large nonstick skillet with the olive oil and preheat over medium-high heat. Add the scallops and cook for about 2 minutes or until nicely browned on the bottoms. Spray the tops lightly with the cooking spray, and turn the scallops over. Cover and cook for an additional 2 minutes or until golden brown and opaque in the center. Serve hot with a squeeze of lemon.

Nutritional Facts (per serving)
Calories: 182   Carbohydrate: 6 g   Cholesterol: 47 mg   Fat: 5.6 g   Saturated Fat: 0.7 g   Fiber: 0.8 g   Protein: 24 g   Sodium: 431 mg   Calcium: 35 mg

Seared Citrus Scallops

✦ FOR A LOVELY PRESENTATION, SERVE THESE SCALLOPS OVER A BED OF LIGHTLY SAUTÉED FRESH SPINACH.

Yield: 4 servings

1¼ pounds large scallops, rinsed and patted dry
1 to 1¼ teaspoons lemon pepper
½ teaspoon garlic powder
¼ teaspoon dried thyme
¼ teaspoon salt

1 tablespoon plus 1 teaspoon extra-virgin olive oil

½ cup orange juice

2 tablespoons finely chopped parsley

1. Place the scallops in a large bowl. Add the lemon pepper, garlic powder, thyme, and salt, and toss to coat. Set aside.

2. Coat a large nonstick skillet with the olive oil and preheat over medium-high heat. Add the scallops and cook for about 2 minutes or until nicely browned on the bottoms. Turn the scallops over, and cook for an additional 2 minutes or until golden brown and opaque in the center. Remove from the skillet and set aside to keep warm.

3. Add the orange juice to the skillet and cook for a minute or two, or until the juice is reduced by half. Divide the scallops between 4 serving plates, drizzle each serving with some of the sauce, and top with a sprinkling of parsley. Serve hot.

Nutritional Facts (per serving)

Calories: 180   Carbohydrate: 6 g   Cholesterol: 47 mg   Fat: 5.6 g   Saturated Fat: 0.7 g   Fiber: 0.1 g   Protein: 24 g   Sodium: 489 mg   Calcium: 40 mg

Fish Fillets Florentine

Yield: 4 servings

4 whitefish fillets such as orange roughy or cod (5 ounces each)

1 teaspoon lemon pepper

½ teaspoon dried oregano

1 tablespoon plus 1 teaspoon extra-virgin olive oil

VEGETABLE MIXTURE

1½ cups sliced fresh mushrooms

¼ cup coarsely shredded carrot, or matchstick-size pieces red bell pepper

3 tablespoons dry white wine or vegetable broth

1 to 2 teaspoons fresh or jarred minced garlic

⅛ teaspoon salt

6 cups (moderately packed) coarsely chopped fresh spinach

1. Rinse the fish fillets with cool water and pat dry with paper towels. Sprinkle both sides of each fillet with some of the lemon pepper and oregano.

2. Coat a large nonstick skillet with the olive oil and preheat over medium-high heat. Add the fish and cook for about 2 to 3 minutes on each side, or until the fish turns opaque and flakes easily with a fork. Remove the fish from the skillet and set aside to keep warm.

3. Add the mushrooms, carrot or red bell pepper, wine or broth, garlic, and salt to the skillet. Cover and cook over medium-high heat for a couple of minutes, until the vegetables start to soften. Add the spinach, and cook uncovered, tossing constantly, for another minute or until the spinach is wilted.

4. Place a quarter of the spinach mixture on each of 4 serving plates, and top the spinach mixture with a fish fillet. Serve hot.

Nutritional Facts (per serving)

Calories: 165   Carbohydrate: 4 g   Cholesterol: 28 mg   Fat: 5.7 g   Saturated Fat: 0.6 g   Fiber: 1 g   Protein: 23 g   Sodium: 315 mg   Calcium: 91 mg

Spicy Grouper with Peppers & Onions

Yield: 4 servings

4 grouper fillets (5 ounces each)
1 tablespoon Cajun Spice Rub (page 76) or Cajun seasoning
1 tablespoon plus 1 teaspoon extra-virgin olive oil

PEPPER MIXTURE
1 medium yellow onion, cut into thin wedges
1 medium green bell pepper, cut into thin strips
1 medium red, yellow, or orange bell pepper, cut into thin strips
¼ cup dry white wine or vegetable broth
¼ teaspoon Cajun Spice Rub (page 76) or Cajun seasoning

1. Rinse the fillets with cool water and pat dry with paper towels. Sprinkle both sides of each fish fillet with some of the Cajun seasoning.

2. Coat a large nonstick skillet with the olive oil and preheat over medium-high heat. Add the fish and cook for about 4 minutes on each side, or until

the fish turns opaque and flakes easily with a fork. Remove the fish from the skillet and set aside to keep warm.

3. Add the onions, bell peppers, wine or broth, and Cajun seasoning to the skillet. Cover and cook over medium-high heat for several minutes or until the vegetables are tender. Add a little more wine if the skillet starts to dry out, but only enough to prevent scorching.
4. Place a fish fillet on each of 4 serving plates and top each fillet with a quarter of the vegetable mixture. Serve hot.

Nutritional Facts (per serving)

*Calories: 199   Carbohydrate: 5 g   Cholesterol: 52 mg   Fat: 5 g   Saturated Fat: 1 g
Fiber: 1.2 g   Protein: 28 g   Sodium: 344 mg   Calcium: 52 mg*

Broiled Fish with Pesto

Yield: 4 servings

4 fish fillets (5 ounces each) such as orange roughy, cod, flounder,
   or salmon
Olive-oil cooking spray
3 to 4 tablespoons prepared pesto
Lemon wedges (garnish)

1. Preheat the broiler. Rinse the fillets and pat dry with paper towels.
2. Coat a broiler pan with cooking spray and lay the fillets on the pan. Spray the fillets lightly with cooking spray. Broil for about 4 minutes or until the tops are nicely browned. Turn the fillets, spread some of the pesto over each one, and broil for an additional 4 minutes or until the fish turns opaque and flakes easily with a fork. Serve hot with lemon wedges.

Nutritional Facts (per serving)

*Calories: 155   Carbohydrate: 5 g   Cholesterol: 28 mg   Fat: 5.6 g   Saturated Fat:
0.4 g   Fiber: 0.3 g   Protein: 23 g   Sodium: 178 mg   Calcium: 125 mg*

Roasted Red Pepper Lasagna

Yield: 8 servings

1 pound 95-percent-lean ground beef, or turkey Italian sausage,
   casings removed

26-ounce jar marinara sauce

1 cup roasted red bell peppers, drained and chopped

¾ cup low-sodium vegetable juice cocktail

10 uncooked whole-wheat lasagna noodles (about 8 ounces)

2 cups shredded reduced-fat mozzarella or Monterey Jack cheese

¼ cup grated Parmesan cheese

CHEESE FILLING

15 ounces nonfat or part-skim ricotta cheese

3 tablespoons fat-free egg substitute

1 teaspoon dried parsley

1. Preheat oven to 350 degrees.
2. Coat a large nonstick skillet with cooking spray and add the ground meat. Cook over medium heat, stirring to crumble, until the meat is nicely browned. Stir in the marinara sauce, roasted red peppers, and vegetable juice, and cook for another minute or two, to heat through. Cover the sauce to keep warm, and set aside.
3. To make the cheese filling, place all of the cheese filling ingredients in a medium-size bowl and stir to mix well. Set aside.
4. To assemble the lasagna, coat a 9-by-13-inch baking pan with nonstick cooking spray, and spoon 1¼ cups of the sauce over the bottom of the pan. Lay 5 of the uncooked noodles over the sauce to cover the bottom of the pan, arranging 4 of the noodles lengthwise, slightly overlapping, and 1 noodle crosswise. (You will have to break about 1 inch off the bottom of the crosswise noodle to make it fit in the pan.)
5. Spread all of the cheese filling over the noodles, then top with half of the mozzarella or Monterey Jack cheese, and another 1½ cups of sauce. Finish layering the casserole with the remaining noodles, sauce, and cheese. Sprinkle the Parmesan over the top.

Main Dish Pastabilities

Pasta can be the perfect solution when you need a meal in a matter of minutes—but can you fit pasta into your carb-conscious lifestyle? Absolutely. Pasta naturally has a low glycemic index, so it provides a slow-release, sustained form of energy. And by choosing whole-wheat pasta, you will get much more nutritional bang for your buck. The pasta recipes in this chapter combine moderate portions of whole-wheat pasta with plenty of lean protein and fiber-rich veggies to create well-balanced dishes with only a moderate amount of carbohydrate. To keep your glycemic load low, be sure to pair your pasta with a fresh garden salad instead of high-carb French or Italian bread.

6. Place the baking pan on a large baking sheet (to catch any drips), cover the pan with aluminum foil (first spraying the underside of the foil with cooking spray to prevent sticking), and bake for 45 minutes. Remove the foil and bake for an additional 15 minutes, or until hot and bubbly. Let stand for 20 minutes before cutting into squares and serving.

Nutritional Facts (per serving)

Calories: 355   Carbohydrate: 34 g   Cholesterol: 50 mg   Fat: 8.7 g   Saturated Fat: 4.7 g   Fiber: 3.6 g   Protein: 35 g   Sodium: 617 mg   Calcium: 525 mg

Penne with Italian Sausage & Spring Vegetables

Yield: 5 servings

8 ounces whole-wheat penne or rotini pasta

2 cups fresh asparagus, cut into 1-inch pieces

1 pound turkey Italian sausage, sliced (partially freezing the sausages will make them easier to slice)

2 cups sliced fresh mushrooms

1¼ cups chopped plum tomatoes

2 cups (moderately packed) fresh spinach, sliced

⅓ cup julienned sun-dried tomatoes in olive oil, drained

Grated Parmesan cheese (optional)

1. Cook the pasta according to package directions. Two minutes before the pasta is done, add the asparagus and cook until the asparagus is crisp-tender and the pasta is al dente. Drain the pasta and asparagus (reserving about ¼ cup of the cooking water) and return it to the pot. Cover it to keep it warm, and set it aside.

2. While the pasta is cooking, coat a large deep nonstick skillet with cooking spray and place over medium heat. Add the sausage and cook over medium heat for several minutes or until nicely browned and no longer pink inside.

3. Add the mushrooms to the skillet, cover, and cook for a couple of minutes, or until the mushrooms begin to brown and release their juices. Stir in the plum tomatoes and cook, covered, for an additional 2 minutes or until the tomatoes start to soften. Stir in the spinach and cook, covered, for another minute to wilt the spinach.

4. Add the pasta, asparagus, and sun-dried tomatoes to the skillet mixture and toss over low heat to mix well. Add some of the reserved pasta water to the skillet if the mixture seems too dry. Serve hot, topping each serving with a sprinkling of Parmesan cheese if desired.

Nutritional Facts (per 1⅞-cup serving)

Calories: 331   Carbohydrate: 38 g   Cholesterol: 76 mg   Fat: 10.5 g   Saturated Fat: 2.8 g   Fiber: 6 g   Protein: 25 g   Sodium: 682 mg   Calcium: 46 mg

Peppery Chicken Pasta

Yield: 5 servings

8 ounces whole-wheat penne or rotini pasta

1 pound boneless skinless chicken breast, cut into thin strips

1 teaspoon dried Italian seasoning

¼ teaspoon garlic powder

¼ teaspoon salt

¼ teaspoon ground black pepper

1 tablespoon extra-virgin olive oil

⅔ cup each red, green, and yellow bell pepper strips

1 medium onion cut into thin wedges

14½-ounce can diced tomatoes with Italian seasonings

¼ teaspoon crushed red pepper

½ cup sliced black olives

Grated Parmesan cheese (optional)

1. Cook the pasta according to package directions. Drain the pasta, return it to the pot, and cover it to keep it warm. Set it aside.

2. Toss the chicken with the Italian seasonings, garlic powder, salt, and pepper. Coat a large nonstick skillet with the olive oil and preheat over medium-high heat. Add the chicken and cook for several minutes or until nicely browned and no longer pink inside. Add the peppers and onions to the skillet and cook for several minutes more or until the vegetables are tender.

3. Add the undrained tomatoes, crushed red pepper, and olives to the skillet mixture. Cover and cook over medium heat for a couple of minutes or until heated through.

4. Add the pasta to the skillet mixture and toss over low heat to mix well. Serve hot, topping each serving with a sprinkling of Parmesan cheese if desired.

Nutritional Facts (per 1⅞-cup serving)

Calories: 348   Carbohydrate: 44 g   Cholesterol: 53 mg   Fat: 6 g   Saturated Fat: 1 g
Fiber: 7 g   Protein: 30 g   Sodium: 500 mg   Calcium: 77 mg

12.

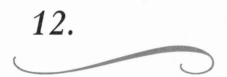

Sensational
Salads

Whether a protein-packed entrée or refreshing side dish, salads are the superstars of a carb-conscious eating plan. Yet people on lower-carb diets can quickly grow weary of salads. This is easy to understand if your salad is a repeat of virtually the same old ingredients day after day. Fortunately, this chapter will prove that there are many simple and creative ways to transform an ordinary salad into extraordinary cuisine.

Beware, though: unless you use the right ingredients, your healthy salad can easily turn into a diet-busting disaster. The fact is, salads piled high with ingredients like full-fat cheeses, fatty meats, and bacon, and drenched with an oily or mayonnaise-y dressing have wrecked the weight-loss goals of many a low-carb devotee. The following recipes will help you sidestep this all-too-common pitfall. As you will see, by combining an assortment of glorious greens and fresh vegetables with lean proteins, low-fat cheeses, and just-right amounts of healthful dressings and other interesting toppings, you can create a dazzling array of satisfying salads that can greatly enhance your dining pleasure.

Menu-Planning Tips

While on the Quick-Start Plan, choose salads made with plenty of fresh leafy greens and raw veggies, lean meats, seafood, skinless poultry, low-fat cheeses, and legumes. Use healthy high-fat foods like nuts and seeds, avocadoes, and oily dressings in moderation, since they are high in calories. A light sprinkling of blue cheese is a fine topper for a salad, since just a little of this flavorful cheese goes a long way.

On the Good-Carb Life Plan, you can expand your selections to enjoy any of the above, plus fruit salads (made with little or no added sweeteners) and moderate portions of salads made with whole-wheat pasta, brown rice, wild, rice, bulgur wheat, barley, and other whole grains. When planning your carb-conscious meals, be sure to balance your entrée with the appropriate side dishes. For instance, if you're having a pasta salad, avoid having other starches in the same meal.

Gorgonzola & Walnut Chicken Salad

Yield: 4 servings

12 cups mixed baby salad greens
½ cup light balsamic vinaigrette salad dressing
2½ cups diced skinless rotisserie chicken, or 4 grilled skinless
    chicken breasts, thinly sliced
⅓ cup julienned sun-dried tomatoes in olive oil, drained
⅓ cup chopped walnuts
⅓ cup crumbled Gorgonzola or blue cheese

1. Place the salad greens in a large bowl. Drizzle with dressing and toss to mix. Divide the salad between 4 large plates.
2. Top the salad greens on each plate with some of the chicken and a sprinkling of tomatoes, walnuts, and cheese. Serve immediately.

Nutritional Facts (per serving)

Calories: 355   Carbohydrate: 12 g   Cholesterol: 83 mg   Fat: 19 g   Saturated Fat: 3.6 g   Fiber: 5 g   Protein: 35 g   Sodium: 567 mg   Calcium: 173 mg

Cancún Chicken Salad

Yield: 4 servings

10 cups mixed baby salad greens

½ cup chopped fresh cilantro

¼ cup plus 2 tablespoons Southwestern Vinaigrette salad dressing
(page 204)

2 cups diced grilled chicken breast or skinless roasted or
rotisserie chicken

1 cup diced avocado

1 cup diced fresh mango

½ cup chopped red onion

⅓ cup coarsely chopped roasted salted cashews

1. Place the salad greens and cilantro in a large bowl. Drizzle with ¼ cup of
   dressing and toss to mix well. Divide the mixture among 4 large plates.
2. Top the salad mixture on each plate with a quarter of the chicken, avocado,
   mangos, onions, and cashews, and drizzle with the remaining dressing. Serve
   immediately.

Nutritional Facts (per serving)

*Calories: 393   Carbohydrate: 22 g   Cholesterol: 62 mg   Fat: 26 g   Saturated Fat: 4 g
Fiber: 6.7 g   Protein: 28 g   Sodium: 366 mg   Calcium: 112 mg*

Southwestern Chicken Chop Salad

Yield: 4 servings

DRESSING

¼ cup extra-virgin olive oil

2 tablespoons white wine vinegar

1 tablespoon honey

1 teaspoon ground cumin

1 to 1½ teaspoons canned chipotle peppers in adobo sauce★

½ teaspoon salt

¼ teaspoon ground black pepper

10 cups chopped romaine lettuce

2 cups diced grilled chicken breast or skinless roasted or
    rotisserie chicken

½ cup black beans, drained and rinsed

½ cup frozen corn, thawed

¾ cup seeded chopped plum tomatoes

½ cup diced orange bell pepper

½ cup chopped red onion

½ cup reduced-fat shredded nonfat or reduced-fat Mexican-
    blend cheese

1. To make the dressing, combine all of the dressing ingredients in a mini
   blender jar and blend to mix well. Set aside.
2. Place the lettuce, chicken, black beans, corn, tomatoes, peppers, and onions
   in a large bowl and toss to mix well. Add the dressing and toss to mix. Add
   the cheese and toss again. Divide the mixture between 4 large plates and
   serve immediately.

Nutritional Facts (per serving)

Calories: 335   Carbohydrate: 23 g   Cholesterol: 51 mg   Fat: 16 g   Saturated Fat:
2.3 g   Fiber: 5.5 g   Protein: 27 g   Sodium: 596 mg   Calcium: 164 mg

---

★ Chipotle chiles in adobo sauce are smoked red jalapeño peppers that are canned in a
tomato-vinegar sauce. Small cans can be found in the Mexican section of most grocery
stores. Leftovers can be frozen in ice-cube trays and transferred to freezer bags for later
use. Be sure to wear gloves when working with all hot peppers as the hot components can
cause a burning sensation.

Asian Chicken & Cabbage Salad

Yield: 4 servings

2 cups shredded skinless roasted or rotisserie chicken

½ cup Soy-Sesame Dressing (page 206)

6 cups coarsely shredded cabbage

2 stalks celery, thinly sliced on the diagonal

½ cup chopped red onion

½ cup chopped fresh cilantro

1 tablespoon toasted sesame seeds

1. Place the chicken and dressing in a large bowl and toss to mix well. Set aside for 5 minutes. Add the cabbage, celery, onion, and cilantro and toss to mix.
2. Serve immediately, topping each serving with some of the sesame seeds, or cover and refrigerate for up to 3 hours before serving.

Nutritional Facts (per serving)

Calories: 277   Carbohydrate: 14 g   Cholesterol: 62 mg   Fat: 13.3 g   Saturated Fat: 2.7 g   Fiber: 3.4 g   Protein: 22.3 g   Sodium: 447 mg   Calcium: 77 mg

Bistro Chicken Salad

Yield: 4 servings

10 cups fresh spinach leaves or mixed baby salad greens

½ cup light balsamic vinaigrette salad dressing

2 cups diced skinless roasted or rotisserie chicken

2 medium pears, cut into thin wedges

¼ cup chopped walnuts

¼ cup dried cherries, cranberries, or golden raisins

¼ cup crumbled reduced-fat feta cheese or blue cheese

1. Place the spinach or mixed greens in a large bowl and toss with half of the salad dressing. Divide the spinach evenly over the bottoms of each of 4 serving plates.
2. Mound a quarter of the chicken in the center of each plate and arrange some of the pear slices around the chicken. Sprinkle each salad with some of the walnuts; cranberries, cherries, or raisins; and cheese. Drizzle each salad with some of the remaining dressing. Serve immediately.

Nutritional Facts (per serving)

Calories: 328   Carbohydrate: 24 g   Cholesterol: 62 mg   Fat: 14 g   Saturated Fat: 1.8 g   Fiber: 3.5 g   Protein: 27 g   Sodium: 487 mg   Calcium: 119 mg

Italian Cobb Salad

Yield: 4 servings

12 cups Italian salad mix or mixed baby salad greens
½ cup light Italian or olive-oil vinaigrette salad dressing
2 cups diced roasted turkey breast, or skinless roasted or
   rotisserie chicken
1 cup diced reduced-fat mozzarella (aged or fresh) or
   provolone cheese
1 cup marinated artichoke hearts, drained and coarsely chopped
1 cup canned garbanzo beans, drained and rinsed
1 cup chopped plum tomatoes
½ cup chopped red onion
⅓ cup sliced black olives
¼ cup shredded Parmesan cheese

1. Place the salad greens and ¼ cup of the dressing in a large bowl, and toss to mix well.
2. Divide the salad mixture evenly over the bottoms of each of 4 plates. Place a quarter of the turkey or chicken in the center of each salad. Arrange a quarter of the mozzarella or provolone, artichoke hearts, garbanzo beans, tomatoes, and onions alongside the turkey or chicken.
3. Drizzle 1 tablespoon of the remaining dressing over each salad, top with some of the olives and Parmesan cheese, and serve immediately.

Nutritional Facts (per serving)
Calories: 392   Carbohydrate: 23 g   Cholesterol: 78 mg   Fat: 18 g   Saturated Fat: 4.7 g   Fiber: 9 g   Protein: 37 g   Sodium: 757 mg   Calcium: 408 mg

Cobb Chop Salad

Yield: 4 servings

10 cups chopped or sliced romaine lettuce
2 cups diced roasted turkey, grilled chicken breast, or skinless
   rotisserie chicken

6 slices turkey bacon, cooked and crumbled

1 cup chopped plum tomato

½ cup crumbled blue cheese

1 cup diced avocado

½ cup chopped red onion

2 hard-boiled eggs, chopped

½ cup plus 2 tablespoons light olive-oil vinaigrette salad dressing

1. Spread the lettuce over the bottom of a large salad bowl. Top with an even layer of the turkey or chicken. Sprinkle the bacon over the top, then continue adding layers of tomatoes, blue cheese, avocado, onion, and egg.
2. Drizzle the dressing over the salad and toss to mix well. Serve immediately.

Nutritional Facts (per serving)

Calories: 392   Carbohydrate: 15 g   Cholesterol: 181 mg   Fat: 22 g   Saturated Fat: 5.1 g   Fiber: 5 g   Protein: 36 g   Sodium: 832 mg   Calcium: 168 mg

Seafood Cobb Salad

Yield: 4 servings

12 cups torn romaine lettuce

½ cup light olive-oil vinaigrette salad dressing

2½ cups steamed shrimp, or cooked crabmeat, or 1¼ cups of each

16 cherry tomatoes, halved

2 cups diced avocado

⅓ cup crumbled blue cheese

4 slices turkey bacon, cooked and crumbled

1. Place the lettuce and salad dressing in a large bowl, and toss to mix well.
2. Arrange a quarter of the lettuce mixture over the bottoms of each of 4 plates. Top each salad with a quarter of the shrimp or crab, tomatoes, avocado, blue cheese, and bacon, and serve immediately.

Nutritional Facts (per serving)

Calories: 362   Carbohydrate: 16 g   Cholesterol: 184 mg   Fat: 23 g   Saturated Fat: 4.5 g   Fiber: 7.4 g   Protein: 28 g   Sodium: 754 mg   Calcium: 165 mg

Chef Salad with Roast Beef & Blue Cheese

Yield: 4 servings

12 cups torn romaine lettuce, spinach, or mixed baby salad greens
20 grape or cherry tomatoes
4 thin slices red onion, separated into rings
½ cup light balsamic vinaigrette salad dressing
12 ounces well-trimmed thinly sliced deli roast beef
¾ cup canned garbanzo beans, rinsed and drained
⅓ cup blue cheese crumbles

1. Combine the salad greens, cherry tomatoes, and onion in a large bowl. Pour the dressing over the top and toss to mix. Divide the salad between 4 large serving plates.
2. Divide the roast beef into 4 stacks. Starting at the long end, roll each stack up into a tight cylinder, and cut crosswise into 1-inch slices. Arrange a quarter of the meat over each salad and sprinkle each salad with some of the garbanzo beans and blue cheese. Serve immediately.

Nutritional Facts (per serving)

Calories: 296   Carbohydrate: 21 g   Cholesterol: 52 mg   Fat: 12.8 g   Saturated Fat: 3.4 g   Fiber: 6.2 g   Protein: 23 g   Sodium: 693 mg   Calcium: 144 mg

Sun-Dried Tomato Chicken Salad

Yield: 4 servings

1½ cups shredded skinless roasted or rotisserie chicken
1 cup chopped canned artichoke hearts, drained
½ cup frozen green peas, thawed
½ cup sliced scallions
⅓ cup julienned sun-dried tomatoes packed in olive oil, drained

DRESSING

1 tablespoon oil from the jar of sun-dried tomatoes

1 tablespoon white wine vinegar

1 tablespoon finely chopped fresh basil, or 1 teaspoon dried basil

¼ teaspoon salt

⅛ teaspoon ground black pepper

1. Combine the chicken, artichoke hearts, peas, scallions, and drained tomatoes in a medium bowl, and toss to mix well.
2. To make the dressing, combine all of the dressing ingredients and stir to mix well. Pour the dressing over the chicken mixture and toss to mix.
3. Let the salad sit for 15 minutes before serving, or cover and chill until ready to serve. If desired, serve on a bed of fresh salad greens garnished with a sprinkling of reduced-fat feta cheese and walnuts, or serve in lettuce-lined pita pockets or whole-wheat wraps.

Nutritional Facts (per ⅞-cup serving)

Calories: 199   Carbohydrate: 15 g   Cholesterol: 45 mg   Fat: 6 g   Sat Fat: 0.6 g Fiber: 6 g   Protein: 21 g   Sodium: 259 mg   Calcium: 56 mg

Southwestern Chicken Salad

Yield: 5 servings

2 cups shredded skinless roasted or rotisserie chicken

1 cup frozen whole kernel corn, thawed

½ cup roasted red bell pepper, drained and chopped

½ cup chopped red or sweet white onion

½ cup finely chopped fresh cilantro

DRESSING

1½ tablespoons extra-virgin olive oil

1½ tablespoons lime juice

2 teaspoons honey

1 teaspoon ground cumin

½ teaspoon chili powder

½ teaspoon salt

¼ teaspoon ground black pepper

1. Combine the chicken, corn, bell peppers, onions, and cilantro in a medium bowl, and toss to mix well.
2. Combine all of the dressing ingredients in a small bowl, and stir to mix well. Pour the dressing over the chicken mixture, and toss to mix well.
3. Let the salad sit for 15 minutes before serving, or cover and chill until ready to serve. If desired, serve on a bed of fresh salad greens or in lettuce-lined pita pockets garnished with avocado slices, or serve wrap-style in whole-wheat flour tortillas lined with mixed salad greens.

Nutritional Facts (per ⅞-cup serving)

Calories: 181   Carbohydrate: 12 g   Cholesterol: 48 mg   Fat: 6.5 g   Saturated Fat: 1.2 g   Fiber: 1.6 g   Protein: 19 g   Sodium: 278 mg   Calcium: 22 mg

Springtime Chicken Salad

Yield: 4 servings

1¼ cups fresh snow peas
2¼ cups shredded skinless roasted or rotisserie chicken
1 medium carrot, shredded with a potato peeler
2 scallions, thinly sliced on the diagonal
1 tablespoon finely chopped fresh dill, or 1 teaspoon dried

DRESSING
1 tablespoon extra-virgin olive oil
1 tablespoon white wine vinegar
1 teaspoon Dijon mustard
1 teaspoon honey
¼ teaspoon salt

1. Fill a 2-quart pot with water and bring to a boil. Add the snow peas and cook for 1 minute, or until crisp-tender. Drain the snow peas, rinse with cool water, and bias slice into thin slivers.
2. Place the snow peas in a bowl, add the chicken, carrot, scallions, and dill, and toss to mix well.
3. Combine all of the dressing ingredients in a small bowl and stir to mix well. Pour the dressing over the chicken mixture, and toss to mix well.

4. Let the salad sit for 15 minutes before serving, or cover and chill until ready to serve. If desired, serve on a bed of fresh salad greens or in whole-wheat pita pockets or whole-wheat wraps lined with mixed salad greens.

Nutritional Facts (per ¾-cup serving)

Calories: 186 Carbohydrate: 5 g Cholesterol: 68 mg Fat: 6.4 g Saturated Fat: 1.3 g Fiber: 1.1 g Protein: 26 g Sodium: 248 mg Calcium: 37 mg

Cilantro Shrimp Salad

Yield: 4 servings

3 cups peeled and de-veined cooked shrimp
⅓ cup finely chopped red onion
¼ cup finely chopped green bell pepper
¼ cup finely chopped red bell pepper
¼ cup finely chopped orange or yellow bell pepper
¼ to ⅓ cup finely chopped fresh cilantro
2 tablespoons extra-virgin olive oil
1 tablespoon lime juice
¼ teaspoon salt
¼ teaspoon ground black pepper

1. Combine the shrimp, onions, peppers, and cilantro in a medium bowl and toss to mix.
2. Drizzle with the olive oil and lime juice, sprinkle with the salt and pepper, and toss again to mix well. Chill for at least 1 hour before serving.

Nutritional Facts (per 1-cup serving)

Calories: 179 Carbohydrate: 3 g Cholesterol: 207 mg Fat: 8 g Saturated Fat: 1.2 g Fiber: 0.8 g Protein: 23 g Sodium: 384 mg Calcium: 48 mg

Raspberry-Walnut Garden Salad

Yield: 4 servings

6 cups mixed baby salad greens

¼ cup Raspberry-Walnut Vinaigrette (page 207)

1 cup fresh raspberries

¼ cup crumbled reduced-fat feta cheese or blue cheese

¼ cup chopped walnuts

1. Place the salad greens and vinaigrette in a large bowl and toss to mix well. Divide the mixture between 4 serving plates.
2. Top each salad with some of the raspberries, cheese, and walnuts, and serve immediately.

Nutritional Facts (per serving)

Calories: 135   Carbohydrate: 7 g   Cholesterol: 0 mg   Fat: 11 g   Saturated Fat: 1.4 g
Fiber: 2.9 g   Protein: 4 g   Sodium: 221 mg   Calcium: 44 mg

Colorful Coleslaw

Yield: 4 servings

1 cup thinly sliced green cabbage

1 cup thinly sliced red cabbage

1 medium carrot shredded with a potato peeler, or ½ cup precut matchstick carrots

DRESSING

1 tablespoon white wine vinegar

1 tablespoon extra-virgin olive oil or canola oil

1 teaspoon honey

1 teaspoon Dijon mustard

½ teaspoon dried dill

¼ teaspoon salt

⅛ teaspoon ground black pepper

1. Place the cabbage and carrots in a medium bowl, and toss to mix.
2. Combine the dressing ingredients in a small bowl and whisk to mix well. Pour the dressing over the salad and toss again. Serve immediately or cover and chill until ready to serve.

Nutritional Facts (per ⅔-cup serving)

Calories: 52   Carbohydrate: 5 g   Cholesterol: 0 mg   Fat: 3.6 g   Saturated Fat: 0.5 g
Fiber: 1.2 g   Protein: 0.8 g   Sodium: 187 mg   Calcium: 25 mg

Spinach Salad Caprese

Yield: 4 servings

6 cups fresh baby spinach
12 cherry tomatoes, halved
¼ cup chopped fresh basil
4 ounces fresh or aged part-skim mozzarella cheese, diced
¼ cup light olive-oil vinaigrette salad dressing

1. Combine the spinach, tomatoes, basil, and mozzarella.
2. Drizzle the dressing over the salad and toss to mix. Serve immediately.

Nutritional Facts (per serving)

Calories: 131   Carbohydrate: 6 g   Cholesterol: 22 mg   Fat: 9.4 g   Saturated Fat: 4 g
Fiber: 1 g   Protein: 7 g   Sodium: 199 mg   Calcium: 211 mg

Sunshine Spinach Salad

Yield: 4 servings

6 cups fresh spinach leaves
4 thin slices red onion, separated into rings
3 to 4 tablespoons Dijon-Dill Dressing (page 205)
1 can (11 ounces) mandarin oranges, well drained
1 small avocado, peeled and sliced
2 tablespoons sliced toasted almonds or roasted salted
   sunflower seeds

1. Place the spinach and onion in a large bowl. Drizzle the dressing over the mixture, and toss to mix well.
2. Arrange a quarter of the spinach mixture on each of 4 serving plates. Arrange a quarter of the orange segments and avocado slices over each salad. Top each salad with a sprinkling of almonds or sunflower seeds, and serve immediately.

Nutritional Facts (per serving)

Calories: 152   Carbohydrate: 14 g   Cholesterol: 0 mg   Fat: 10.7 g   Saturated Fat: 1 g   Fiber: 4.1 g   Protein: 3.2 g   Sodium: 128 mg   Calcium: 65 mg

Roasted Beet Salad with Blue Cheese & Walnuts

Yield: 4 servings

3 medium beets (each about 2½ inches diameter)
¼ cup Dijon-Dill Dressing (page 205)
6 cups (moderately packed) fresh spinach
1 cup fresh orange segments, or 1 can (11 ounces) Mandarin
   orange segments, drained
¼ cup chopped red onion
3 tablespoons chopped walnuts
3 tablespoons crumbled blue cheese

1. Leave the rootlets and 1 inch of the stems on the beets, and scrub well. Wrap the beets together in aluminum foil and place on a medium baking sheet. Bake at 400 degrees for about 1 hour, or until the beets are easily pierced with a toothpick. Open the foil, and allow the beets to cool to room temperature.
2. Peel the beets, cut into thin strips, and toss with 1 tablespoon of the dressing. Cover and refrigerate for at least 1 hour or until ready to assemble the salad. (You can prepare the beets the day before if desired.)
3. To assemble the salads, place the spinach in a large bowl, and add the remaining dressing. Toss to mix well and divide the mixture between 4 salad plates. Top each salad with a quarter of the beet mixture and arrange a

quarter of the orange segments around the beets on each salad. Sprinkle each salad with some of the onions, walnuts, and blue cheese, and serve immediately.

Nutritional Facts (per serving)

Calories: 176   Carbohydrate: 14 g   Cholesterol: 5 mg   Fat: 12 g   Saturated Fat: 2.3 g   Fiber: 3.5 g   Protein: 4.4 g   Sodium: 251 mg   Calcium: 70 mg

Carrot-Pecan Salad

Yield: 4 servings

2 cups coarsely shredded carrots
¼ cup chopped toasted pecans (page 240)
2 tablespoons finely chopped fresh parsley, or 2 teaspoons dried

DRESSING
1 tablespoon canola oil
1 tablespoon lemon juice
1 teaspoon honey
⅛ teaspoon salt

1. Combine the carrots, pecans, and parsley in a medium bowl, and toss to mix well. Combine the canola oil, lemon juice, honey, and salt in a small bowl, and stir to mix well.
2. Pour the dressing over the salad and toss to mix well. Serve immediately or cover and refrigerate until ready to serve.

Nutritional Facts (per ½-cup serving)

Calories: 112   Carbohydrate: 8 g   Cholesterol: 0 mg   Fat: 8.8 g   Saturated Fat: 0.7 g   Fiber: 2.4 g   Protein: 1.3 g   Sodium: 93 mg   Calcium: 23 mg

Green Bean & Tomato Salad

Yield: 8 servings

5 cups 1-inch pieces fresh green beans (about 1 pound)

1 cup seeded and diced plum tomatoes

½ cup chopped red onion

2 tablespoons finely chopped fresh dill, or 2 teaspoons dried

DRESSING

¼ cup white balsamic vinegar, or ¼ cup white wine vinegar plus
  2 teaspoons honey

2 tablespoons extra virgin olive oil

1 teaspoon fresh or jarred minced garlic

Scant ½ teaspoon salt

¼ teaspoon ground black pepper

1. Cook the green beans in boiling water for about 4 minutes, or until crisp-tender. Drain the beans, rinse with cool water, and drain again. Place the beans, tomatoes, onions, and dill in a shallow bowl and toss to mix well.
2. Combine all of the dressing ingredients in a small bowl and stir to mix well. Pour the dressing over the green-bean mixture and toss to mix well. Cover and chill for several hours, stirring occasionally, before serving.

Nutritional Facts (per ⅔-cup serving)

Calories: 59   Carbohydrate: 7 g   Cholesterol: 0 mg   Fat: 3.5 g   Saturated Fat: 0.5 g   Fiber: 2.1 g   Protein: 1.2 g   Sodium: 115 mg   Calcium: 24 mg

Guacamole Salad

Yield: 4 servings

2½ cups diced peeled avocado

1½ teaspoons lime juice

¼ cup chopped seeded plum tomato

2 tablespoons finely chopped onion

2 tablespoons finely chopped cilantro

½ teaspoon fresh or jarred minced garlic

¼ teaspoon salt

2 cups shredded romaine lettuce

1. Place the avocado in a medium bowl and mash with a fork, leaving the mixture slightly chunky. Stir in the lime juice, tomato, onion, cilantro, garlic, and salt.

2. Place ½ cup of the lettuce on each of 4 salad plates and top the lettuce on each plate with a quarter of the avocado mixture. Serve immediately.

Nutritional Facts (per serving)

Calories: 159   Carbohydrate: 9 g   Cholesterol: 0 mg   Fat: 14 g   Saturated Fat: 2.3 g

Fiber: 5.4 g   Protein: 2.5 g   Sodium: 159 mg   Calcium: 23 mg

Roasted Pepper Salad

Yield: 4 servings

1 medium-large red bell pepper, cut into ¾-inch thick strips

1 medium-large green bell pepper, cut into ¾-inch thick strips

1 medium-large yellow bell pepper, cut into ¾-inch thick strips

Olive-oil cooking spray

¼ teaspoon Italian seasoning

3 tablespoons light balsamic vinaigrette salad dressing

3 tablespoons crumbled reduced-fat feta cheese

1. Preheat oven to 450 degrees. Coat a 9-by-13-inch pan with cooking spray and place the peppers in the pan. Spray the peppers lightly with the cooking spray and sprinkle with the Italian seasoning.

2. Bake for 10 minutes. Stir the mixture and cook for an additional 12 minutes, stirring a couple of times or until the peppers are tender and nicely browned. Let the peppers cool to room temperature.

3. Place the peppers in a medium bowl, add the salad dressing, and toss to mix well. Serve immediately, or cover and chill until ready to serve. Bring the pepper mixture to room temperature before serving. Top with the feta cheese just before serving.

Nutritional Facts (per ½-cup serving)

Calories: 58   Carbohydrate: 7 g   Cholesterol: 2 mg   Fat: 2.8 g   Saturated Fat: 0.5 g

Fiber: 1.7 g   Protein: 1.9 g   Sodium: 180 mg   Calcium: 23 mg

Broccoli–Barley Salad

Yield: 8 servings

3 cups cooked barley

1½ cups chopped broccoli florets and diced peeled stems
  (about ⅓-inch pieces)

¾ cup grated carrots

⅓ cup thinly sliced scallions

1 to 2 tablespoons finely chopped fresh dill, or 1 to
  2 teaspoons dried

½ cup chopped toasted pecans (optional)

DRESSING

2 tablespoons extra-virgin olive oil

1 tablespoon plus 1 teaspoon frozen (thawed) orange juice
  concentrate

1 tablespoon plus 1 teaspoon lemon juice

½ teaspoon salt

1. Combine the barley, broccoli, carrots, scallions, dill, and if desired, the pecans in a large bowl, and toss to mix well.
2. Combine the dressing ingredients in a small bowl and whisk to mix well. Pour the dressing over the barley mixture and toss to mix well. Cover the salad and chill for at least 2 hours before serving.

Nutritional Facts (per ¾-cup serving)

*Calories: 168   Carbohydrate: 21 g   Cholesterol: 0 mg   Fat: 9 g   Saturated Fat: 1 g
Fiber: 4 g   Protein: 2.7 g   Sodium: 155 mg   Calcium: 27 mg*

Black-Eyed Pea Salad

Yield: 5 servings

15-ounce can black-eyed peas, rinsed and drained

1 cup frozen whole kernel corn, thawed

¼ cup finely chopped celery

¼ cup finely chopped red bell pepper

¼ cup finely chopped onion

¼ cup chopped fresh cilantro

DRESSING

1 tablespoon extra-virgin olive oil

1 tablespoon white or red wine vinegar

1 teaspoon Dijon or spicy mustard

1 teaspoon honey

½ teaspoon ground cumin

¼ teaspoon salt

1. Combine the black-eyed peas, corn, celery, peppers, onions, and cilantro in a medium bowl, and toss to mix well. Set aside.
2. Combine all of the dressing ingredients in a small bowl, and stir to mix well. Pour the dressing over the salad, and toss to mix well.
3. Cover the salad, and refrigerate for at least 3 hours before serving.

Nutritional Facts (per ⅔-cup serving)

Calories: 131   Carbohydrate: 21 g   Cholesterol: 0 mg   Fat: 3.4 g   Saturated Fat: 0.5 g   Fiber: 5 g   Protein: 5.7 g   Sodium: 254 mg   Calcium: 21 mg

Mediterranean Tuna Pasta Salad

Yield: 6 servings

8 ounces whole-wheat penne or rotini pasta

12-ounce can albacore tuna in water, drained

1½ cups canned chopped artichoke hearts, drained

½ cup sliced black olives

½ cup diagonally sliced scallions

1 cup roasted red bell peppers, drained and chopped

½ cup crumbled reduced-fat feta cheese

DRESSING

¼ cup nonfat or light mayonnaise

¼ cup light olive-oil vinaigrette or Italian salad dressing

1 teaspoon dried basil

¼ teaspoon ground black pepper

1. Cook the pasta al dente according to package directions. Drain well, rinse with cool water, and drain again.
2. Place the pasta, tuna, artichoke hearts, olives, scallions, and half of the roasted red bell peppers in a large bowl, and toss to mix.
3. To make the dressing, place the remaining roasted red bell peppers, mayonnaise, Italian dressing, basil, and pepper in a blender or mini food processor, and process until smooth. Add the dressing to the salad, and toss to mix well.
4. Cover the salad and chill for at least 2 hours before serving. Mix in a little more Italian dressing just before serving if the salad seems too dry. Toss in the feta cheese just before serving. Serve over a bed of fresh spinach or romaine lettuce if desired.

Nutritional Facts (per 1½-cup serving)

Calories: 293   Carbohydrate: 38 g   Cholesterol: 27 mg   Fat: 6.9 g   Saturated Fat: 1.6 g   Fiber: 6.6 g   Protein: 22 g   Sodium: 627 mg   Calcium: 82 mg

Sesame Chicken & Pasta Salad

Yield: 5 servings

6 ounces whole-wheat rotini or penne pasta

1½ cups 1-inch pieces fresh asparagus

2½ cups shredded skinless roasted or rotisserie chicken breast

½ cup matchstick-size pieces red or yellow bell pepper

½ cup sliced scallions

1½ tablespoons toasted sesame seeds

DRESSING

3 tablespoons rice vinegar

3 tablespoons reduced-sodium soy sauce

2 tablespoons toasted sesame oil

2 tablespoons apricot spreadable fruit

½ teaspoon ground ginger, or 1½ teaspoons fresh grated ginger

2 cups fresh spinach leaves, thinly sliced

Dazzling Dressings

A great dressing can make or break a salad, and many fine ready-made dressings are now available in your grocery store. Both light and regular dressings can have places in your carb-conscious eating plan as long as you moderate portions to keep calories under control. If you use a high-quality, intensely flavored dressing, you may be surprised at how little is required to dress a salad. Pages 204–207 present a selection of easy-to-make dressings that are full of fresh-made flavor.

1. Cook the pasta al dente according to package directions. Add the asparagus to the pot and cook for 1 minute more, or until crisp-tender. Drain the pasta and asparagus, rinse with cool water, and drain again.
2. Place the pasta mixture, chicken, bell peppers, scallions, and sesame seeds in a large bowl, and toss to mix. Combine all of the dressing ingredients in a blender and blend until smooth. Pour the dressing over the pasta mixture, and toss to mix.
3. Cover the salad and refrigerate for at least 2 hours. Toss in the spinach just before serving.

Nutritional Facts (per 1⅔-cup serving)

Calories: 336   Carbohydrate: 33 g   Cholesterol: 60 mg   Fat: 8.6 g   Saturated Fat: 1.6 g   Fiber: 4 g   Protein: 29 g   Sodium: 608 mg   Calcium: 53 mg

Southwestern Vinaigrette

Yield: about 1 cup

½ cup extra-virgin olive oil
¼ cup plus 2 tablespoons white wine vinegar
2 tablespoons honey
1 tablespoon Dijon mustard

2 teaspoons ground cumin

1¼ teaspoons chili powder

¾ teaspoon salt

½ teaspoon ground black pepper

1. Combine all of the ingredients in a mini blender jar and blend for 1 minute to mix well.
2. Serve immediately, or cover and refrigerate until ready to use. Shake well before serving.

Nutritional Facts (per tablespoon)

Calories: 65   Carbohydrate: 2 g   Cholesterol: 0 mg   Fat: 6.5 g   Saturated Fat: 0.9 g   Fiber: 0.2 g   Protein: 0.1 g   Sodium: 128 mg   Calcium: 5 mg

Dijon-Dill Dressing

Yield: ¾ cup

¼ cup white wine vinegar

¼ cup plus 2 tablespoons extra-virgin olive oil or walnut oil

1 tablespoon honey

2 teaspoons Dijon mustard

1 teaspoon dried dill

½ teaspoon salt

¼ teaspoon ground black pepper

1. Combine all of the ingredients in a blender and blend for 1 minute to mix well.
2. Serve immediately, or cover and refrigerate until ready to use. Shake well before serving.

Nutritional Facts (per tablespoon)

Calories: 66   Carbohydrate: 1.6 g   Cholesterol: 0 mg   Fat: 6.8 g   Saturated Fat: 0.9 g   Fiber: 0 g   Protein: 0.1 g   Sodium: 118 mg   Calcium: 3 mg

Greek Isle Dressing

Yield: about 1¼ cups

½ cup extra-virgin olive oil
¾ cup crumbled reduced-fat feta cheese
3 tablespoons white wine vinegar
2 tablespoons water
1 tablespoon lemon juice
2 teaspoons honey
1½ teaspoons fresh or jarred minced garlic
½ teaspoon dried oregano
½ teaspoon ground black pepper
Scant ½ teaspoon salt

1. Combine all of the ingredients in a blender and blend until smooth.
2. Serve immediately, or cover and refrigerate until ready to use. Shake well before serving.

Nutritional Facts (per tablespoon)
*Calories: 59   Carbohydrate: 0.7 g   Cholesterol: 1 mg   Fat: 6 g   Saturated Fat: 1.1 g
Fiber: 0 g   Protein: 1 g   Sodium: 106 mg   Calcium: 13 mg*

Soy-Sesame Dressing

Yield: ⅞ cup

¼ cup low-sugar apricot fruit spread
¼ cup rice vinegar
¼ cup sesame oil
2 tablespoons reduced-sodium soy sauce
½ teaspoon ground ginger

1. Combine all of the ingredients in a blender and blend until smooth.
2. Serve immediately, or cover and refrigerate until ready to use. Shake well before serving.

Nutritional Facts (per tablespoon)

*Calories: 40   Carbohydrate: 1.7 g   Cholesterol: 0 mg   Fat: 3.9 g   Saturated Fat: 0.6 g
Fiber: 0 g   Protein: 0 g   Sodium: 128 mg   Calcium: 0 mg*

Raspberry-Walnut Vinaigrette

Yield: about ⅔ cup

¼ cup walnut oil
3 tablespoons light (low-sugar) raspberry preserves
3 tablespoons white wine vinegar
¼ teaspoon dried thyme
½ teaspoon salt
¼ teaspoon ground black pepper

1. Place all of the ingredients in a mini blender jar and blend to mix well.
2. Serve immediately or cover and chill until ready to serve. Shake well before serving.

Nutritional Facts (per 1-tablespoon serving)

*Calories: 54   Carbohydrate: 1.8 g   Cholesterol: 0 mg   Fat: 5.4 g   Saturated Fat: 0.5 g
Fiber: 0 g   Protein: 0 g   Sodium: 117 mg   Calcium: 1 mg*

13.

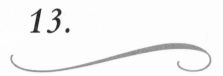

Simply Delicious
Side Dishes

Side dishes present a terrific opportunity to add health-promoting veggies to your meals. And busy cooks will be happy to know that the less you do to vegetables in the way of cooking, the better off your side dishes will be, nutritionally. Simple cooking methods like steaming, roasting, sautéing, and stir-frying are superior techniques for preserving nutrients.

You can also make healthful side dishes from whole grains like brown rice, wild rice, bulgur wheat, barley, quinoa, and whole-wheat couscous. By combining these grains with plenty of garden vegetables, you can create delicious dishes with only a moderate amount of carbohydrate. Add some garlic, herbs, and a little olive oil, and your savory side dishes will be special enough for any occasion.

Menu Planning Tips

While on the Quick-Start Plan, limit your side-dish choices to the low- and medium-carb vegetables listed in Chapter 5. Season your veggies with ingredients like garlic, herbs, a little olive oil, and a light sprinkling of nuts or grated Parmesan cheese. This chapter provides an array of appropriate dishes to get you started.

On the Good-Carb Life Plan you can also enjoy moderate portions of higher-carb side dishes like sweet potatoes, new potatoes, corn on the cob, winter squash, and pilafs made with whole grains. (A list of high-carb vegetables can be found in Chapter 5.) However, when including higher-carb side dishes in meals, be sure to balance the meal out with lower-carb items such as a lean protein entrée and a low-carb garden salad.

Asparagus Amandine

Yield: 2 servings

2 tablespoons sliced almonds
8 ounces young tender asparagus spears (snap off the tough stem
  ends)
1 teaspoon margarine or butter
⅛ teaspoon salt

1. Place the almonds in a large nonstick skillet (do not coat with cooking spray) and place over medium-high heat. Cook for about 30 seconds, shaking the skillet frequently, until the almonds are very lightly browned. Remove the almonds and set aside.
2. Spray the skillet with cooking spray and add the asparagus. Cover and cook over medium-high heat for about 4 minutes, shaking the pan frequently, until the asparagus are crisp-tender and lightly browned.
3. Reduce the heat to low, add the margarine or butter, and shake the pan until the margarine or butter melts and coats the asparagus. Sprinkle the almonds over the top, shake the pan again, and serve hot.

Nutritional Facts (per serving)
*Calories: 78   Carbohydrate: 6 g   Cholesterol: 0 mg   Fat: 4.8 g   Saturated Fat: 0.7 g
Fiber: 3.6 g   Protein: 3.6 g   Sodium: 162 mg   Calcium: 36 mg*

Easy Baked Brussels Sprouts

Yield: 5 servings

1 pound frozen Brussels sprouts
¼ teaspoon salt
¼ teaspoon dried dill or thyme
1 tablespoon extra-virgin olive oil

1. Preheat the oven to 400 degrees.
2. Coat a 9-by-13-inch pan with cooking spray, and place the frozen Brussels sprouts in the dish. Sprinkle with the salt and herbs. Drizzle with the olive oil, and toss to mix well.
3. Cover the pan with aluminum foil and bake for about 25 minutes, or until steaming hot and tender. Serve immediately.

Nutritional Facts (per ⅔-cup serving)
Calories: 61   Carbohydrate: 7 g   Cholesterol: 0 mg   Fat: 2.9 g   Saturated Fat: 0.4 g   Fiber: 3.5 g   Protein: 3 g   Sodium: 125 mg   Calcium: 24 mg

Green Beans with Walnuts

Yield: 6 servings

5 cups of 1-inch pieces fresh green beans (about 1¼ pounds)
1 tablespoon walnut oil or canola oil
3 tablespoons finely chopped walnuts
¼ teaspoon salt
½ teaspoon dried dill

1. Cook the green beans in boiling water for 4 minutes or until crisp-tender. Drain well and return to the pot.
2. Drizzle the walnut oil over the green beans and sprinkle with the walnuts, salt, and dill. Toss to mix well. Serve hot.

Nutritional Facts (per ⅔-cup serving)
Calories: 72   Carbohydrate: 6 g   Cholesterol: 0 mg   Fat: 4.7 g   Saturated Fat: 0.4 g   Fiber: 3 g   Protein: 1.7 g   Sodium: 96 mg   Calcium: 48 mg

Broccoli with Garlic & Olive Oil

Yield: 5 servings

4½ cups fresh broccoli florets and coarsely chopped stems
¼ cup water
1 tablespoon extra-virgin olive oil
1½ teaspoons fresh or jarred minced garlic
¼ teaspoon salt
Grated Parmesan cheese (optional)

1. Coat a large nonstick skillet with cooking spray and place over medium-high heat. Add the broccoli and water. Cover and cook, stirring occasionally, for several minutes, or until the broccoli is crisp-tender. Add a little more water if the skillet becomes too dry, but only enough to prevent scorching.
2. Drain any excess liquid from the skillet. Push the broccoli to one side of the skillet, and add the olive oil and garlic to the other. Cook for about 10 seconds, or until the garlic begins to turn color and smell fragrant. Toss the broccoli with the garlic and olive oil. Add the salt and toss to mix well. Serve hot, topping each serving with some Parmesan cheese if desired.

Nutritional Facts (per ¾-cup serving)
*Calories: 43   Carbohydrate: 4 g   Cholesterol: 0 mg   Fat: 2.9 g   Saturated Fat: 0.4 g
Fiber: 2.1 g   Protein: 2 g   Sodium: 133 mg   Calcium: 34 mg*

Caraway Cabbage

Yield: 4 servings

½ large head cabbage, cored
⅛ to ¼ teaspoon caraway seeds
⅛ teaspoon salt
½ cup unsalted chicken or vegetable broth
2 teaspoons extra-virgin olive oil

1. Cut the piece of cabbage in half and then into ¼-inch slices. Place the cabbage in a large nonstick skillet and sprinkle with the caraway seeds and salt. Pour the broth over the top.

2. Cover and cook over medium heat for about 15 minutes, stirring occasionally, until the cabbage is tender. If necessary, cook uncovered for a few minutes to evaporate any excess liquid. Toss in the olive oil and serve hot.

Nutritional Facts (per ¾-cup serving)

Calories: 49   Carbohydrate: 4 g   Cholesterol: 0 mg   Fat: 2.5 g   Saturated Fat: 0.3 g   Fiber: 2.6 g   Protein: 1.7 g   Sodium: 93 mg   Calcium: 54 mg

Rosemary Roasted Carrots

Yield: 5 servings

1 pound baby carrots
¾ teaspoon dried rosemary, crumbled
¼ teaspoon garlic powder
¼ teaspoon salt
1 tablespoon extra-virgin olive oil

1. Preheat the oven to 425 degrees.
2. Place the carrots in an 8-by-8-inch baking pan and sprinkle with the rosemary, garlic powder, and salt. Drizzle with the olive oil and toss to mix.
3. Bake uncovered for about 25 minutes, stirring after 15 minutes, until the carrots are tender and nicely browned. Serve hot.

Nutritional Facts (per ½-cup serving)

Calories: 58   Carbohydrate: 7 g   Cholesterol: 0 mg   Fat: 3.2 g   Saturated Fat: 0.5 g   Fiber: 2 g   Protein: 1 g   Sodium: 148 mg   Calcium: 23 mg

Cauliflower with Fresh Herbs

Yield: 5 servings

5 cups fresh cauliflower florets
½ cup water
Scant ¼ teaspoon salt
1 tablespoon extra-virgin olive oil or walnut oil

1 tablespoon finely chopped fresh parsley, or 1 teaspoon dried
1 tablespoon finely chopped fresh dill, or 1 teaspoon dried

1. Place the cauliflower, water, and salt in a large nonstick skillet, and place over medium-high heat. Cover and cook for 6 to 8 minutes or until tender. (Add a little water during cooking if needed, but only enough to prevent scorching.)
2. Remove the skillet from the heat and drain off any excess water. Add the oil and herbs, and toss to mix well. Serve hot.

Nutritional Facts (per ¾-cup serving)

*Calories: 49   Carbohydrate: 5 g   Cholesterol: 0 mg   Fat: 2.9 g   Saturated Fat: 0.2 g
Fiber: 2.6 g   Protein: 2 g   Sodium: 123 mg   Calcium: 25 mg*

Savory Collard Greens

Yield: 5 servings

1 tablespoon canola or olive oil
½ cup chopped yellow onion
1 teaspoon fresh or jarred minced garlic
1 pound frozen chopped collard greens
1 cup water
¼ teaspoon salt

1. Place the oil in a 3-quart nonstick pot and add the onions. Cover and cook over medium heat for several minutes, or until the onions start to soften. Add the garlic and cook for a few seconds more, or just until the garlic begins to turn color and smell fragrant.
2. Add the greens, water, and salt, and bring the mixture to a boil. Reduce the heat to low, cover, and simmer for 20 to 25 minutes, or until the greens are tender. Serve hot. Top each serving with a dash of hot sauce if desired.

Nutritional Facts (per ⅔-cup serving)

*Calories: 60   Carbohydrate: 7 g   Cholesterol: 0 mg   Fat: 2.9 g   Saturated Fat: 0.2 g
Fiber: 2.5 g   Protein: 2.6 g   Sodium: 157 mg   Calcium: 173 mg*

Spring Vegetable Medley

Yield: 5 servings

2 cups fresh cauliflower florets, sliced ½-inch thick
2 cups fresh 1-inch broccoli florets
1 cup ¼-inch thick diagonally sliced carrots
1 tablespoon canola or olive oil
1 teaspoon dried dill or parsley
⅛ teaspoon salt

1. Preheat the oven to 400 degrees.
2. Place the vegetables in a 9-by-13-inch nonstick pan. Drizzle with the oil, sprinkle with the herbs and salt, and toss to mix well.
3. Cover the pan with aluminum foil and bake for about 20 minutes, or until tender. Serve hot.

Nutritional Facts (per ¾-cup serving)
Calories: 45   Carbohydrate: 5 g   Cholesterol: 0 mg   Fat: 2.8 g   Saturated Fat: 0.4 g   Fiber: 2 g   Protein: 1.1 g   Sodium: 79 mg   Calcium: 16 mg

Broiled Rosemary Mushrooms

Yield: 4 servings

1 pound (about 6 cups) fresh mushrooms, sliced
½ teaspoon dried rosemary
¼ teaspoon salt
¼ teaspoon ground black pepper
1 tablespoon extra virgin olive oil

1. Place the mushrooms, rosemary, salt, and pepper in a large bowl. Drizzle the oil over the top and toss to mix well.
2. Coat a large nonstick baking sheet with cooking spray and spread the mush-

rooms evenly over the pan. Broil for about 8 minutes, stirring several times until the mushrooms are tender and lightly browned. Serve hot.

Nutritional Facts (per ½-cup serving)

Calories: 58   Carbohydrate: 5 g   Cholesterol: 0 mg   Fat: 3.7 g   Saturated Fat: 0.5 g

Fiber: 1.4 g   Protein: 3.3 g   Sodium: 149 mg   Calcium: 7 mg

Stuffed Portobello Mushrooms

Yield: 4 servings

4 medium-large portobello mushrooms
2 teaspoons extra-virgin olive oil
½ cup chopped celery
½ cup chopped red bell pepper
½ cup sliced scallions
¾ teaspoon dried oregano
1 teaspoon fresh or jarred minced garlic
2 medium-small plum tomatoes, seeded and chopped
¾ cup prepared bulgur wheat or whole-wheat couscous
3 tablespoons grated Parmesan cheese
Olive oil cooking spray

1. Preheat the oven to 450 degrees.
2. Trim the stems from the mushrooms and use a spoon to scrape out the gills, creating a shallow depression in each mushroom. Set aside.
3. Coat a large nonstick skillet with the olive oil and add the celery, peppers, scallions, and oregano. Cover and cook over medium heat for several minutes, stirring occasionally, or until the vegetables are tender. Add the garlic and tomatoes, and cook for another minute or until the tomatoes are soft. Remove the skillet from the heat and stir in the bulgur wheat or couscous and Parmesan cheese.
4. Mound a quarter of the vegetable mixture in the depression of each mushroom cap. Spray the tops lightly with cooking spray. Place the mushrooms

on a baking sheet and bake uncovered at 450 degrees for 15 minutes or until the mushrooms are tender and the topping is lightly browned. Serve hot.

Nutritional Facts (per serving)

*Calories: 96   Carbohydrate: 12 g   Cholesterol: 3 mg   Fat: 3.9 g   Saturated Fat: 1.2 g
Fiber: 3.5 g   Protein: 4.8 g   Sodium: 108 mg   Calcium: 93 mg*

Tricolored Pepper Sauté

Yield: 5 servings

1 tablespoon extra-virgin olive oil
1 medium green bell pepper, cut into thin strips
1 medium red bell pepper, cut into thin strips
1 medium yellow bell pepper, cut into thin strips
1 medium yellow onion, cut into thin wedges
½ teaspoon dried oregano or thyme
¼ teaspoon salt
¼ teaspoon ground black pepper
1 teaspoon fresh or jarred minced garlic

1. Coat a large nonstick skillet with the olive oil and add the remaining ingredients except the garlic. Place the skillet over medium-high heat. Cover and cook for several minutes, stirring several times, or until the vegetables start to soften.
2. Reduce the heat to medium, add the garlic, and continue to cook, covered, for a few minutes more, or until the vegetables are tender. Serve hot.

Nutritional Facts (per ½-cup serving)

*Calories: 50   Carbohydrate: 6 g   Cholesterol: 0 mg   Fat: 2.9 g   Saturated Fat: 0.4 g
Fiber: 2 g   Protein: 1 g   Sodium: 118 mg   Calcium: 11 mg*

Spaghetti Squash with Pesto

Yield: 8 servings

2-pound spaghetti squash
¼ cup prepared pesto

1. Preheat the oven to 375 degrees.
2. Rinse the squash, cut it in half lengthwise, and scoop out the seeds. Coat a large baking sheet with cooking spray and lay the squash halves, cut-side down, on the sheet. Bake for about 45 minutes, or until the squash can be easily pierced with a fork.
3. Cut each squash half into quarters. Spoon 1½ teaspoons of pesto over each piece and use a fork to fluff the center of each piece of squash slightly and mix in the pesto. Serve hot.

Nutritional Facts (per serving)
Calories: 63   Carbohydrate: 6 g   Cholesterol: 2 mg   Fat: 3.8 g   Saturated Fat: 1 g
Fiber: 1.6 g   Protein: 2 g   Sodium: 76 mg   Calcium: 74 mg

Sesame Spinach

Yield: 4 servings

10-ounce package prewashed fresh baby spinach (about 10 cups)
1 tablespoon sesame oil
1 tablespoon reduced-sodium soy sauce

1. Coat a large deep skillet with nonstick cooking spray. Add the spinach to the skillet and drizzle with the sesame oil and soy sauce.
2. Cook over medium heat, tossing gently, for a couple of minutes, or until the spinach is wilted. Serve hot.

Nutritional Facts (per ⅔-cup serving)
Calories: 48   Carbohydrate: 3 g   Cholesterol: 0 mg   Fat: 3.6 g   Saturated Fat: 0.5 g
Fiber: 1.8 g   Protein: 2.3 g   Sodium: 207 mg   Calcium: 70 mg

Herb-Roasted Potatoes, Onions, & Mushrooms

Yield: 7 servings

1 pound new potatoes, cut into ¾-inch chunks

8 ounces medium whole fresh mushrooms, halved

2 medium yellow onions, cut into 1-inch wedges

2 tablespoons extra-virgin olive oil

2 teaspoons Dijon mustard

1 teaspoon dried rosemary

¼ teaspoon salt

⅛ teaspoon ground black pepper

1. Preheat the oven to 450 degrees.
2. Place all of the vegetables in a large bowl and toss to mix well. Combine the olive oil, mustard, rosemary, salt, and pepper, and drizzle over the vegetables. Toss to mix.
3. Coat an 11-by-13-inch nonstick roasting pan or the bottom of a large broiler pan with cooking spray, and spread the vegetable mixture over the bottom of the pan.
4. Bake for 10 minutes, stir the vegetables, and cook for an additional 20 minutes, stirring every 5 minutes, or until the vegetables are tender and nicely browned. Serve hot.

Nutritional Facts (per ¾-cup serving)

Calories: 112   Carbohydrate: 18 g   Cholesterol: 0 mg   Fat: 3.9 g   Saturated Fat: 0.4 g   Fiber: 2.1 g   Protein: 2.4 g   Sodium: 116 mg   Calcium: 14 mg

Roasted Zucchini, Peppers, & Onions

Yield: 5 servings

3 medium zucchini squash, sliced (about 3 cups)

1 medium red bell pepper, cut into 1-inch strips

2 medium-small yellow onions, cut into rings

¾ teaspoon dried Italian seasoning

¼ teaspoon garlic powder

⅛ teaspoon ground black pepper

¼ teaspoon salt

1 tablespoon extra-virgin olive oil

1. Preheat oven to 450 degrees.
2. Place all of the ingredients in a large bowl and toss to mix. Coat an 11-by-13-inch roasting pan or the bottom of a broiler pan with cooking spray and spread the vegetables over the bottom of the pan.
3. Bake for 15 minutes. Stir the vegetables and cook for another 5 to 10 minutes, or until they are tender and nicely browned. Serve hot.

Nutritional Facts (per ⅔-cup serving)

*Calories: 55   Carbohydrate: 7 g   Cholesterol: 0 mg   Fat: 2.9 g   Saturated Fat: 0.4 g
Fiber: 2.1 g   Protein: 1.5 g   Sodium: 120 mg   Calcium: 21 mg*

Zucchini Pomodoro

Yield: 5 servings

1 tablespoon extra-virgin olive oil

1 teaspoon fresh or jarred minced garlic

4 medium zucchini squash, halved lengthwise and sliced

½ teaspoon dried basil

¼ teaspoon salt

¼ teaspoon ground black pepper

4 medium-small plum tomatoes, seeded and diced

1. Coat a large nonstick skillet with the olive oil. Add the garlic, squash, basil, salt, and pepper, and sauté over medium-high heat for several minutes, or until the zucchini are crisp-tender.
2. Add the tomatoes and cook for another minute or two, or until the tomatoes are heated through and start to soften. Serve immediately.

Nutritional Facts (per ¾-cup serving)

*Calories: 49   Carbohydrate: 9 g   Cholesterol: 0 mg   Fat: 3 g   Saturated Fat: 0.4 g
Fiber: 2 g   Protein: 1.8 g   Sodium: 123 mg   Calcium: 21 mg*

Pilaf with Zucchini & Sun-Dried Tomatoes

Yield: 7 servings

2 to 3 tablespoons sun-dried tomatoes in olive oil and Italian
    seasonings, drained and chopped, plus 1 tablespoon of oil
    from the jar of sun-dried tomatoes
½ cup chopped yellow onion
1½ cups ⅓-inch diced zucchini
1 teaspoon fresh or jarred minced garlic
3 cups cooked brown rice (or 1½ cups brown rice plus 1½ cups
    wild rice), or prepared bulgur wheat
Scant ½ teaspoon salt
⅛ teaspoon ground black pepper
2 tablespoons finely chopped fresh parsley

1. Coat a large nonstick skillet with the oil from the jar of sun-dried tomatoes
    and preheat over medium heat. Add the onion, cover, and cook for a cou-
    ple of minutes or until the onions start to soften. Add the zucchini and cook
    for another minute or two, or just until the zucchini is crisp-tender. Add the
    garlic and cook for another few seconds or just until the garlic begins to turn
    color and smell fragrant.
2. Add the rice, salt, and pepper to the skillet, and toss over medium heat for a
    minute or two to heat through. Toss in the parsley and serve hot.

Nutritional Facts (per ⅔-cup serving)
*Calories: 121   Carbohydrate: 21 g   Cholesterol: 0 mg   Fat: 3 g   Saturated Fat: 0.5 g
Fiber: 2.1 g   Protein: 2.6 g   Sodium: 144 mg   Calcium: 16 mg*

Spring Vegetable Pilaf

Yield: 7 servings

1 tablespoon extra-virgin olive oil
½ cup chopped yellow onion

1 teaspoon dried savory or fines herbes

1 cup ¾-inch pieces fresh asparagus spears (use thin spears for
  best results)

½ cup diced red bell pepper

½ cup frozen green peas, thawed

1 teaspoon fresh or jarred minced garlic

3 cups cooked brown rice (or 1½ cups brown rice plus 1½ cups
  wild rice)

Scant ½ teaspoon salt

⅛ teaspoon ground black pepper

1. Coat a large nonstick skillet with the olive oil and preheat over medium heat. Add the onion and savory or fines herbes, cover, and cook for a couple of minutes or until the onions start to soften. Add the asparagus and bell pepper and cook for another minute or two, or until the vegetables are crisp-tender. Add the peas and garlic, and cook for another few seconds or until the garlic begins to turn color and smell fragrant.
2. Add the rice, salt, and pepper to the skillet and toss over medium heat for a minute or two to heat through. Serve hot.

Nutritional Facts (per ⅔-cup serving)

Calories: 129   Carbohydrate: 23 g   Cholesterol: 0 mg   Fat: 2.8 g   Saturated Fat: 0.4 g   Fiber: 2.8 g   Protein: 3.6 g   Sodium: 149 mg   Calcium: 18 mg

Bulgur Pilaf with Sautéed Spinach & Onions

Yield: 7 servings

1 tablespoon extra-virgin olive oil

½ cup finely chopped onion

½ cup finely chopped yellow bell pepper

¾ teaspoon ground cumin

6 cups (moderately packed) fresh spinach, thinly sliced

1 teaspoon fresh or jarred minced garlic

3 cups prepared bulgur wheat

Scant ½ teaspoon salt

⅛ teaspoon ground black pepper

¼ cup pine nuts (optional)

1. Coat a large nonstick skillet with the olive oil and preheat over medium heat. Add the onion, bell pepper, and cumin. Cover and cook for a couple of minutes or until the vegetables are tender. Add the spinach and garlic and cook for another minute or two, or until the spinach wilts.

2. Add the bulgur wheat, salt, pepper, and if desired, the pine nuts to the skillet, and toss over medium heat for a minute or two to heat through. Serve hot.

Nutritional Facts (per ⅔-cup serving)

Calories: 117   Carbohydrate: 21 g   Cholesterol: 0 mg   Fat: 2.5 g   Saturated Fat: 0.4 g   Fiber: 5 g   Protein: 3 g   Sodium: 156 mg   Calcium: 36 mg

14.

Smart
Sandwiches

Perhaps the most longed-for fare on a low-carb diet is
the simple sandwich. Hence, the proliferation of extreme versions of
high-protein, low-carb bread—products that often fall short on satis-
faction. The good news is that going to extreme measures with bread
and giving up sandwiches as a life-long weight-control strategy is just
plain silly and unnecessary. That said, there's a big difference between a
sandwich made with supersize white bread and one made with a right-
size whole-grain alternative. Filled with lean protein and piled high
with fresh veggies, a sandwich can be a satisfying part of your carb-
conscious lifestyle. Many people have also discovered the ultra light
"lettuce wrap"—which features savory sandwich fillings enclosed in a
fresh lettuce leaf.

Realize, too, that what you have *with* your sandwich can make or
break your meal. Keep your carbohydrate load down by choosing a garden salad, cup of soup, or fresh fruit instead of starchy accompaniments
like chips, fries, and pretzels.

This chapter offers a selection of hearty and creative sandwiches
that are a snap to make. Whether you are looking for an original wrap,

a satisfying burger, or a garden-style sandwich sans bread, you are sure to find a sandwich that meets your need deliciously.

Menu-Planning Tips

While on the Quick-Start Plan, limit your choices to lettuce wrap–style sandwiches. Choose from any of the lettuce wraps in this chapter or create your own concoction filled with your favorite light tuna salad, chicken salad, hummus, and other lean protein and veggie fillings.

On the Good-Carb Life Plan, you may enjoy any of the above, plus sandwiches made with whole-grain pitas, whole-wheat wraps, and whole-grain breads and burger buns. If you like, you can cut carbs by using light or reduced-carb versions of breads and buns. Some of these products are very good, while others more closely resemble cardboard! So experiment to see which ones you like best. Rest assured, there is no problem with eating whole-grain versions of the "real thing" as long as you keep portions in perspective.

Turkey & Artichoke Lettuce Wraps

Yield: 4 wraps

4 large Boston lettuce leaves
6 ounces thinly sliced turkey
2 ounces thinly sliced reduced-fat Swiss cheese
⅓ cup marinated artichoke hearts, drained and chopped
1 tablespoon plus 1 teaspoon nonfat or light mayonnaise

1. Lay the lettuce leaves on a flat surface with the stem ends facing you. Layer a quarter of the turkey and cheese on the lower portion of each leaf. Combine the artichoke hearts and mayonnaise, and spread a quarter of the mixture over each wrap.
2. Roll the leaves up to enclose the filling. Secure with a toothpick and serve immediately.

Nutritional Facts (per wrap)

Calories: 107   Carbohydrate: 2 g   Cholesterol: 40 mg   Fat: 3 g   Saturated Fat: 1.2 g
Fiber: 1.1 g   Protein: 18 g   Sodium: 215 mg   Calcium: 137 mg

Roast Beef & Roasted Pepper Lettuce Wraps

Yield: 4 wraps

4 large Boston lettuce leaves

6 ounces thinly sliced roast beef

2 ounces thinly sliced reduced-fat mozzarella or provolone cheese

1½ tablespoons nonfat or light mayonnaise

4 strips roasted red bell pepper

2 very thin slices red onion, separated into rings

1. Lay the lettuce leaves on a flat surface with the stem ends facing you. Layer a quarter of the roast beef and cheese on the lower portion of each leaf. Spread some of the mayonnaise over the cheese layer, and top with a strip of red bell pepper and some of the onion.
2. Roll the leaves up to enclose the filling. Secure with a toothpick and serve immediately.

Nutritional Facts (per wrap)

Calories: 106   Carbohydrate: 3 g   Cholesterol: 31 mg   Fat: 3.6 g   Saturated Fat: 1.8 g   Fiber: 0.6 g   Protein: 14 g   Sodium: 295 mg   Calcium: 130 mg

Ham & Cheese Lettuce Wraps

Yield: 4 wraps

4 large Boston lettuce leaves

6 ounces thinly sliced lean reduced-sodium ham

2 ounces thinly sliced reduced-fat Swiss cheese

1½ tablespoons nonfat or light mayonnaise

1 teaspoon Dijon mustard

8 thin slices plum tomato

1. Lay the lettuce leaves on a flat surface with the stem ends facing you. Layer a quarter of the ham and cheese on the lower portion of each leaf.

2. Combine the mayonnaise and mustard, and spread some of the mixture over the cheese on each wrap. Top each piece with a couple of tomato slices and roll the leaves up to enclose the filling. Secure with a toothpick and serve immediately.

Nutritional Facts (per wrap)

Calories: 90   Carbohydrate: 4 g   Cholesterol: 16 mg   Fat: 3.1 g   Saturated Fat: 1.4 g Fiber: 0.3 g   Protein: 12 g   Sodium: 340 mg   Calcium: 131 mg

Cashew Chicken Salad Lettuce Wraps

Yield: 6 wraps

1½ cups shredded skinless roasted or rotisserie chicken
⅓ cup chopped roasted cashews
¼ cup finely chopped celery
3 tablespoons thinly sliced scallions
3 tablespoons finely chopped red bell pepper
⅓ cup nonfat or light mayonnaise
6 large leaves Boston lettuce

1. Combine the chicken, cashews, celery, scallions, and bell peppers, and toss to mix. Stir in the mayonnaise.
2. Lay the lettuce leaves on a flat surface with the stem ends facing you. Spread about ⅓ cup of the chicken salad on the lower portion of each leaf. Roll the leaves up to enclose the filling, secure with a toothpick, and serve immediately.

Nutritional Facts (per wrap)

Calories: 115   Carbohydrate: 5 g   Cholesterol: 30 mg   Fat: 4.8 g   Saturated Fat: 1 g Fiber: 0.6 g   Protein: 12 g   Sodium: 172 mg   Calcium: 16 mg

West Coast Lettuce Wraps

Yield: 4 wraps

4 large Boston lettuce leaves
6 ounces thinly sliced turkey or chicken breast

Making Low-Carb Lettuce Wrap Sandwiches.

You can trim carbs from many of your favorite sandwiches by making them into lettuce wraps. Instead of bread, wrap your favorite sandwich filling in a pliable leaf of lettuce such as Boston or leaf lettuce. Lay a large lettuce leaf on a flat surface with the stem end facing you. Lay the sandwich fillings on the lower portion of the leaf, and roll the leaf up to enclose the filling.

2 ounces thinly sliced reduced-fat Swiss or Monterey Jack cheese
8 thin slices avocado
1½ tablespoons light ranch or blue cheese salad dressing
2 very thin slices red onion, separated into rings

1. Lay the lettuce leaves on a flat surface with the stem ends facing you. Layer a quarter of the turkey, cheese, and avocado slices on the lower portion of each leaf.
2. Spread some of the dressing over each wrap and top with some of the onion rings. Roll the leaves up to enclose the filling. Secure with a toothpick and serve immediately.

Nutritional Facts (per wrap)
Calories: 128   Carbohydrate: 3 g   Cholesterol: 42 mg   Fat: 4.9 g   Saturated Fat: 1.5 g   Fiber: 0.8 g   Protein: 18 g   Sodium: 151 mg   Calcium: 139 mg

California Chicken Pitas

Yield: 4 servings

3½ cups torn romaine lettuce
¾ cup diced avocado
½ cup coarsely shredded purple cabbage
2 slices red onion, separated into rings

8 ounces grilled or roasted chicken, diced

¼ cup light olive-oil vinaigrette or ranch salad dressing

4 whole-wheat or oat-bran pita pockets (6-inch rounds),
cut in half

1. Place the lettuce, avocado, cabbage, onion, and chicken in a large bowl, and toss to mix well. Add the salad dressing and toss again. Set aside.
2. To heat the pita pockets, place them on a microwave-safe plate. Cover with a damp paper towel, and microwave on high power for about 45 seconds, or until warm. If heating only one pita at a time, microwave for only 20 seconds.
3. To assemble the sandwiches, place about ¾ cup of the lettuce mixture in each of the 8 pita halves, and serve immediately.

Nutritional Facts (per serving)

Calories: 308   Carbohydrate: 39 g   Cholesterol: 40 mg   Fat: 9.5 g   Saturated Fat: 1 g
Fiber: 7 g   Protein: 22 g   Sodium: 621 mg   Calcium: 69 mg

Dilly Tuna Salad Sandwiches

Yield: 4 servings

12-ounce can tuna in water, drained

⅓ cup grated carrots

⅓ cup finely chopped celery

¼ cup thinly sliced scallions

¼ to ⅓ cup nonfat or light mayonnaise

1 teaspoon dried dill

8 slices firm whole-wheat or multigrain bread

4 lettuce leaves

1. Place the tuna, carrots, celery, and scallions in a medium bowl, and toss to mix well. Add half of the mayonnaise and the dill, and toss to mix well. Mix in a little more mayonnaise if the mixture seems too dry.
2. To assemble the sandwiches, toast the bread if desired, and spread each piece with some of the remaining mayonnaise. Place one-fourth of the tuna salad mixture on the bottom half of each bread slice, and top with a lettuce leaf.

3. Place the top halves of the bread slices on the sandwiches, cut each sandwich in half, and serve immediately.

Nutritional Facts (per serving)

Calories: 283   Carbohydrate: 31 g   Cholesterol: 25 mg   Fat: 3.7 g   Saturated Fat: 0.2 g   Fiber: 5 g   Protein: 29 g   Sodium: 611 mg   Calcium: 20 mg

Cheesy Crab Melts

Yield: 4 servings

1½ cups cooked crabmeat, or 2 cans (6 ounces each) crabmeat, drained
½ cup finely chopped celery
⅓ cup finely chopped sweet onion
¼ cup finely chopped red bell pepper
⅓ cup nonfat or light mayonnaise
1½ teaspoons Dijon mustard
¼ teaspoon dried dill
4 whole-wheat or oat-bran English muffins, split and toasted
1 cup shredded reduced-fat Swiss or Havarti cheese

1. Combine the crabmeat, celery, onions, and bell peppers in a medium bowl, and toss to mix well. Combine the mayonnaise, mustard, and dill in a small bowl, and stir to mix well. Add the mayonnaise mixture to the crab mixture and toss to mix well.
2. Arrange the English muffins on a baking sheet, split-side up. Spread about ¼ cup of the crab mixture over each piece and place under a preheated broiler for 2 to 3 minutes, or until the crab mixture is heated through. Top each muffin half with 2 tablespoons of the cheese, and broil for another minute or two or until the cheese is melted. Serve hot.

Nutritional Facts (per serving)

Calories: 275   Carbohydrate: 31 g   Cholesterol: 55 mg   Fat: 5.9 g   Saturated Fat: 2.4 g   Fiber: 5 g   Protein: 24 g   Sodium: 875 mg   Calcium: 486 mg

Greek Hamburgers

Yield: 5 servings

1 pound 95-percent-lean ground beef or turkey

1 cup finely chopped fresh mushrooms

½ cup finely chopped onion

1 teaspoon dried rosemary

½ teaspoon garlic powder

½ teaspoon ground black pepper

¼ teaspoon salt

¼ cup nonfat or light mayonnaise

1 tablespoon plus 1 teaspoon Dijon mustard

5 whole-wheat or oat-bran pita pocket halves

25 large fresh spinach leaves

5 slices roasted red bell pepper

⅓ cup crumbled reduced-fat feta cheese with sun-dried
   tomatoes and herbs

1. Place the ground beef or turkey, mushrooms, onion, rosemary, garlic powder, black pepper, and salt in a medium bowl, and mix thoroughly. Shape the
mixture into five patties.

2. Grill the burgers over medium coals or cook under a broiler for about 6
minutes on each side, or until the internal temperature of the patties reaches
160 degrees for ground beef, or 165 degrees for ground turkey, and the meat
is no longer pink inside. Alternatively, coat a large nonstick skillet or griddle
with nonstick cooking spray, and cook the burgers over medium heat for
about 5 minutes per side. (To retain moisture, avoid pressing down on the
patties as they cook.)

3. Combine the mayonnaise and mustard and mix well. Spread some of the
mixture in each of the pita pockets and line with the spinach leaves. Place
each burger in a pita pocket and top with some of the red bell pepper and
feta cheese. Serve hot.

Nutritional Facts (per serving)
*Calories: 223   Carbohydrate: 20 g   Cholesterol: 52 mg   Fat: 5.8 g   Saturated Fat:
2.4 g   Fiber: 3 g   Protein: 24 g   Sodium: 611 mg   Calcium: 59 mg*

Burgers Dijon

Yield: 6 servings

BURGER MIXTURE
1¼ cups sliced fresh mushrooms
½ cup chopped onion
⅓ cup chopped celery
1¼ pounds 95-percent-lean ground turkey or beef
2 tablespoons Dijon mustard
2 tablespoons finely chopped fresh parsley, or 2 teaspoons dried
¼ teaspoon ground black pepper

6 whole-wheat or multigrain burger buns
6 slices tomato
6 slices red onion
6 lettuce leaves

1. Place the mushrooms, onion, and celery in the bowl of a food processor and process until the vegetables are finely chopped. Place the vegetables, ground turkey or beef, mustard, parsley, and black pepper in a medium bowl, and mix thoroughly. Shape the mixture into six 4-inch patties.
2. Grill the burgers over medium coals or cook under a broiler for about 6 minutes on each side, or until the internal temperature of the patties reaches 160 degrees or 165 degrees for turkey and the meat is no longer pink inside. Alternatively, coat a large nonstick skillet or griddle with cooking spray, and cook the burgers over medium heat for about 5 minutes per side. (To retain moisture, avoid pressing down on the patties as they cook.)
3. Place each burger in a bun and top with some of the tomatoes, onions, and lettuce, and your choice of condiments. Serve hot.

Nutritional Facts (per serving)
Calories: 271   Carbohydrate: 25 g   Cholesterol: 58 mg   Fat: 6.7 g   Saturated Fat: 0.7 g   Fiber: 5 g   Protein: 27 g   Sodium: 384 mg   Calcium: 63 mg

Pesto Turkey Wraps

Yield: 4 servings

4 whole-wheat flour tortillas (8- to 9-inch rounds), brought to
  room temperature
2 to 3 tablespoons prepared pesto
2 tablespoons nonfat or light mayonnaise
8 ounces thinly sliced roasted turkey breast
4 slices (¾ ounce each) reduced-fat provolone or
  mozzarella cheese
1 medium plum tomato, thinly sliced
12 large fresh spinach leaves

1. Lay the tortillas out on a flat surface and spread each one with a quarter of the pesto and mayonnaise.
2. Top the *bottom half only* of each tortilla with a quarter of the turkey, cheese, tomato slices, and spinach, leaving a 1½-inch margin on the right and left sides.
3. Fold the right and left margins in, then roll each tortilla up from the bottom to enclose the filling. Place the wraps on a microwave-safe plate and cover with a paper towel. Microwave at high power for about 1½ minutes, or until warmed through. (If heating only 1 wrap at a time, microwave for about 30 seconds.) Cut each wrap in half and serve immediately.

Nutritional Facts (per serving)

Calories: 326   Carbohydrate: 28 g   Cholesterol: 49 mg   Fat: 10.4 g   Saturated Fat: 1 g   Fiber: 2.6 g   Protein: 29 g   Sodium: 646 mg   Calcium: 230 mg

California Club Wraps

Yield: 4 servings

4 whole-wheat flour tortillas (8- to 10-inch rounds)
½ cup light vegetable-flavored cream cheese
6 ounces thinly sliced roasted turkey breast
4 slices cooked turkey bacon

8 slices avocado

2 slices red onion, separated into rings

16 fresh spinach leaves, or 1 cup alfalfa sprouts

1. Warm the tortillas according to package directions. Lay the tortillas on a flat surface, and spread each one with 2 tablespoons of the cream cheese, extending the cream cheese to within 1-inch of the edges.

2. Top the *bottom half only* of each tortilla with a quarter of the turkey, 1 bacon slice, 2 slices of avocado, a quarter of the onion rings, and a quarter of the spinach leaves or sprouts, leaving a 1½-inch margin on the right and left sides.

3. Fold the right and left margins in, then roll each tortilla up from the bottom, jellyroll style. Cut each wrap in half and serve immediately.

Nutritional Facts (per serving)

Calories: 322   Carbohydrates: 32 g   Cholesterol: 72 mg   Fat: 11 g   Saturated Fat: 4 g   Fiber: 4.4 g   Protein: 23 g   Sodium: 692 mg   Calcium: 94 mg

15.

Something for the Sweet Tooth

Living a lower-carb lifestyle does not necessarily mean giving up dessert. Having said that, moderation is still the best policy when it comes to sweets—and some desserts are definitely better choices than others. And do be aware that the "sugar-free" and "low-carb" desserts featured in some lower-carb cookbooks and restaurants may deliver much more than you bargained for. Cups of heavy cream, gobs of butter and full-fat cream cheese, and other fatty ingredients can quickly turn a sweet treat into an artery-clogging, calorie-laden diet buster!

The reduced-carb recipes in this chapter feature lighter, more wholesome ingredients, and can be enjoyed as part of your Good-Carb Life Plan. Healthful oils, lower-fat dairy products, naturally sweet fruits, nuts, and whole grains are combined with moderate amounts of sugar and low-cal sweeteners to create a dazzling array of deceptively decadent desserts. Whether you are looking for an almond-crusted fruit pie, a creamy cherry-topped cheesecake, or a moist mocha-fudge cake, here you will find many delicious ways to satisfy a sweet tooth.

Menu-Planning Tips

If you opt for the Low-Carb Quick-Start Plan, you will temporarily give up sweets and desserts. But once you progress to the Good-Carb Life Plan, you can occasionally indulge in a sweet treat. Having said that, personal philosophies on eating sugar vary greatly. Some people believe that they fare much better by avoiding sweets entirely. Others find that completely depriving themselves can backfire by leading to unhealthy food obsessions and binge eating. The bottom line is that different approaches work for different people, so experiment to find the right balance for you.

Sensational Strawberry Pie

Yield: 8 servings

CRUST
Unbleached flour (about 1 tablespoon)
1¼ cups sliced almonds
2 tablespoons sugar
Pinch salt
Sugar substitute equal to 2 tablespoons sugar
1½ teaspoons fat-free egg substitute

5 cups halved fresh strawberries
1½ cups sugar-free strawberry glaze
1 cup nonfat or light whipped topping (optional)

1. Preheat oven to 350 degrees.
2. To make the crust, line a 9-inch pie pan with heavy-duty aluminum foil and spray with cooking spray. Lightly dust with the flour, shaking out the excess. Set aside.
3. Place the almonds, sugar, and salt in a food processor and process until finely ground. Add the sugar substitute and egg substitute and process for a few seconds more or until the mixture is moist and crumbly and holds together when pinched.
4. Press the almond mixture over the bottom and sides of the pan. (Place your

hand inside a small plastic bag as you press, to prevent sticking.) Bake for about 8 minutes or until the crust feels firm and dry and is lightly browned. Cool to room temperature, then peel away and discard the aluminum foil. Place the crust back in the pan. (Note: You can make the crust the day before and cover with foil until ready to use.)

5. Combine the berries and glaze in a large bowl and toss to mix. Pile the mixture into the crust. Cover and refrigerate for 2 to 5 hours before serving. Top each serving with some of the whipped topping if desired.

Nutritional Facts (per serving)

Calories: 146 Carbohydrate: 16 g Cholesterol: 0 mg Fat: 8.7 g Saturated Fat: 0.7 g Fiber: 3.9 g Protein: 4.3 g Sodium: 67 mg Calcium: 49 mg

Cheesecake Supreme

Yield: 12 servings

2 tablespoons graham cracker crumbs
1 cup part-skim ricotta cheese
¾ cup sugar
Sugar substitute equal to ½ cup sugar
2 teaspoons vanilla extract
3 blocks (8 ounces each) light (Neufchâtel) cream cheese,
  softened to room temperature
1 tablespoon cornstarch
3 eggs
20-ounce can no-added-sugar or light cherry-pie filling, or 1 can
  light apple-pie filling, chopped

1. Preheat oven to 325 degrees.
2. Coat a 9-inch springform pan with cooking spray and sprinkle the graham cracker crumbs over the bottom of the pan. Tilt the pan so the crumbs coat the bottom and 1 inch up the sides of the pan. Set aside.
3. Place the ricotta, ½ cup plus 2 tablespoons of the sugar, all of the sugar substitute, and vanilla in a large bowl and beat to mix well. Add the cream cheese and beat until smooth. Sprinkle the cornstarch over the top and beat to mix well.

4. Add 2 of the eggs plus 1 yolk to the cream cheese mixture and beat to mix well. Place the remaining egg white in a medium bowl. Wash off the beaters, and then beat the egg white until soft peaks form. Slowly add the remaining 2 tablespoons of sugar and beat until stiff peaks form when the beaters are raised. Fold the whipped egg white into the cheesecake batter.
5. Spread the batter evenly in the prepared pan. Wrap a piece of heavy-duty aluminum foil over the bottom and up the sides of the pan (to prevent any leaks). Bake for about 55 minutes, or just until the center feels firm to the touch. Let the cake cool to room temperature.
6. Spread the pie filling over the cake and chill for at least 8 hours or overnight before serving.

Nutritional Facts (per serving)

*Calories: 264   Carbohydrate: 21 g   Cholesterol: 100 mg   Fat: 15 g   Saturated Fat: 9 g
Fiber: 0.3 g   Protein: 10 g   Sodium: 300 mg   Calcium: 103 mg*

Cinnamon-Apple Cake

Yield: 9 servings

½ cup unbleached flour
½ cup whole-wheat pastry flour or oat flour
⅔ cup brown sugar
1½ teaspoons ground cinnamon
½ teaspoon baking soda
¼ cup fat-free egg substitute, or 1 egg, lightly beaten
3 tablespoons walnut or canola oil
2 tablespoons nonfat or low-fat milk
1 teaspoon vanilla extract
2 cups grated or very finely chopped peeled Granny Smith apples
   (about 3 medium)
⅓ cup chopped walnuts
⅓ cup dark raisins (optional)

1. Preheat the oven to 350 degrees.
2. Place the flours, brown sugar, cinnamon, and baking soda in a medium bowl, and stir to mix well. Use the back of a spoon to press out the lumps

in the brown sugar. Combine the egg substitute or eggs, oil, milk, and vanilla extract, and stir to mix well. Add the egg mixture and apples to the flour mixture and stir just until the dry ingredients are moistened. Set the batter aside for 10 minutes.

3. Add the nuts, and if desired the raisins, and stir to mix well. Coat an 8-inch square pan with cooking spray and spread the batter evenly in the pan.

4. Bake for about 30 minutes, or until the top springs back when lightly touched and a wooden toothpick inserted in the center of the cake comes out clean. Let the cake cool to room temperature before cutting into squares and serving.

Nutritional Facts (per serving)

Calories: 151   Carbohydrate: 31 g   Cholesterol: 0 mg   Fat: 7.3 g   Saturated Fat: 0.5 g   Fiber: 2 g   Protein: 3.6 g   Sodium: 98 mg   Calcium: 24 mg

Fudge Cake with Fresh Berries

Yield: 9 servings

½ cup unbleached flour

½ cup oat flour

⅓ cup cocoa powder (preferably Dutch-process cocoa)

½ cup sugar

Sugar substitute equal to ⅓ cup sugar

⅛ teaspoon ground cinnamon

½ teaspoon baking soda

Scant ¼ teaspoon salt

¾ cup room-temperature coffee

¼ cup canola or walnut oil

2 tablespoons fat-free egg substitute, or 1 egg white, lightly beaten

1 teaspoon vanilla extract

TOPPINGS

2¼ cups sliced strawberries or fresh raspberries

½ cup light (reduced-sugar) chocolate syrup

1 cup plus 2 tablespoons nonfat or light whipped topping

1. Preheat the oven to 350 degrees.
2. Place the flours, cocoa powder, sugar, sugar substitute, cinnamon, baking soda, and salt in a large bowl and whisk to mix well. Combine the coffee, oil, egg substitute or egg white, and vanilla extract in a small bowl, and stir to mix well. Add the coffee mixture to the flour mixture and whisk to mix well.
3. Set the batter aside for 10 minutes, and then whisk for 10 more seconds. Coat an 8-by-8-inch pan with cooking spray and spread the batter evenly in the pan.
4. Bake at 350 degrees for about 25 minutes, or until a wooden toothpick inserted in the center of the cake comes out clean or coated with a few fudgy crumbs. Let the cake cool to room temperature.
5. Cut the cake into squares and top each piece with ¼ cup of the berries and some of the chocolate syrup and whipped topping.

Nutritional Facts (per serving)

*Calories: 200   Carbohydrate: 33 g   Cholesterol: 0 mg   Fat: 7 g   Saturated Fat: 0.6 g
Fiber: 2.5 g   Protein: 3.2 g   Sodium: 152 mg   Calcium: 15 mg*

Pear & Pecan Crisp

Yield: 8 servings

2 cans (15 ounces each) sliced pears in juice
2½ teaspoons cornstarch
Sugar substitute equal to 3 to 4 tablespoons sugar

TOPPING
½ cup old-fashioned (5-minute) oats
2 tablespoons whole-wheat pastry flour
¼ cup plus 2 tablespoons light brown sugar
¾ teaspoon ground cinnamon
½ teaspoon ground ginger
2 tablespoons soft reduced-fat margarine
½ cup chopped toasted pecans (page 240)

1. Preheat the oven to 375 degrees F.
2. Drain the pears reserving ½ cup of the juice. Place the cornstarch in a

2-quart pot, add a tablespoon of the reserved juice, and stir to dissolve the cornstarch. Stir in the remaining reserved juice. Bring the mixture to a boil over medium-high heat. Cook and stir for a minute or two or until the juice has thickened. Stir in the sugar substitute and pears and heat through.

3. Coat a 9-inch pie pan with cooking spray and spread the pear mixture evenly in the dish.

4. To make the topping, place the oats, flour, brown sugar, cinnamon, and ginger in a medium bowl and stir to mix well. Add the margarine and stir until the mixture is moist and crumbly. Add a little more margarine if the mixture seems too dry. Stir in the nuts.

5. Sprinkle the topping over the fruit and bake, uncovered, for about 20 minutes or until the filling is bubbly around the edges and the topping is golden brown. Let sit for 20 minutes before serving.

Nutritional Facts (per serving)

*Calories: 172   Carbohydrate: 27 g   Cholesterol: 0 mg   Fat: 7 g   Saturated Fat: 0.9 g
Fiber: 2.6 g   Protein: 2 g   Sodium: 32 mg   Calcium: 23 mg*

Toasting Nuts

Nuts make a deliciously crunchy addition to all kinds of recipes. And by lightly toasting them, you can bring out their deep, rich flavors even more, and transform a dish from ordinary into extraordinary. To toast nuts, simply arrange the desired amount in a single layer on a baking sheet and bake at 350 degrees until lightly browned with a toasted, nutty aroma. Chopped or sliced nuts will be done in as little as five minutes, while whole or halved nuts will take a little longer. Just be careful to watch them closely during the last part of baking as they can become burned very quickly. To save time, toast some extras and store leftovers in the freezer or refrigerator.

Berries & Cream

Yield: 4 servings

½ cup light sour cream
1 tablespoon nonfat or low-fat milk
Sugar substitute equal to 2 tablespoons sugar
1 cup nonfat or light whipped topping
1⅓ cups fresh raspberries, rinsed and patted dry
1⅓ cups fresh blackberries or blueberries, rinsed and patted dry
2 tablespoons sliced almonds

1. Combine the sour cream, milk, and sugar substitute in a small bowl and stir to mix well. Fold in the whipped topping.
2. Mix the berries together and place ⅓ cup in each of four 8-ounce wine glasses. Top with 3 tablespoons of the sour cream mixture. Repeat the layers and top each serving with a sprinkling of almonds. Serve immediately.

Nutritional Facts (per serving)
Calories: 126   Carbohydrates: 23 g   Cholesterol: 0 mg   Fat: 2.7 g   Saturated Fat: 0.5 g   Fiber: 5.6 g   Protein: 3.4 g   Sodium: 35 mg   Calcium: 72 mg

Lemon-Berry Parfait

Yield: 4 servings

1 cup light lemon yogurt
½ cup nonfat or light whipped topping
2 cups fresh blueberries or blackberries, rinsed and patted dry

1. Place the yogurt in a bowl and fold in the whipped topping.
2. Place ¼ cup of berries in each of four 8-ounce wine glasses. Top the berries in each glass with 3 tablespoons of the lemon yogurt mixture. Repeat the layers, and serve immediately.

Nutritional Facts (per serving)
Calories: 83   Carbohydrate: 17 g   Cholesterol: 1 mg   Fat: 0.6 g   Saturated Fat: 0 g   Fiber: 2 g   Protein: 3 g   Sodium: 44 mg   Calcium: 80 mg

Chocolate-Raspberry Parfait

Yield: 4 servings

2 cups fresh raspberries, rinsed and patted dry

¼ cup light (reduced-sugar) chocolate syrup

1 cup nonfat or light whipped topping

2 tablespoons sliced almonds

Place ¼ cup of raspberries in each of four 8-ounce wine glasses. Top the berries in each glass with ½ tablespoon of the chocolate syrup and 2 tablespoons of whipped topping. Repeat the layers, and then top each serving with a sprinkling of almonds. Serve immediately.

Nutritional Facts (per serving)

Calories: 104   Carbohydrates: 20 g   Cholesterol: 0 mg   Fat: 2.6 g   Saturated Fat: 0.1 g   Fiber: 4.5 g   Protein: 2 g   Sodium: 23 mg   Calcium: 21 mg

Cherry Pudding Parfait

Yield: 4 servings

1 package (4-serving size) sugar-free instant vanilla, chocolate, or white-chocolate pudding mix

2 cups nonfat or low-fat milk

1 cup no-sugar-added or light (reduced-sugar) cherry-pie filling

½ cup nonfat or light whipped topping

1½ tablespoons shaved or finely chopped dark chocolate

1. Place the pudding mix and milk in a large bowl and whisk for 2 minutes or until well mixed and thickened.

2. Place ¼ cup of the pudding in each of four 8-ounce wine glasses. Top the pudding in each glass with 2 tablespoons of the pie filling. Repeat the layers. Cover and chill for at least 1 hour before serving. Top each serving

with a dollop of whipped topping and a sprinkling of chocolate just before serving.

Nutritional Facts (per ¾-cup serving)

Calories: 138   Carbohydrate: 26 g   Cholesterol: 2 mg   Fat: 1.7 g   Saturated Fat: 0.8 g   Fiber: 1 g   Protein: 4 g   Sodium: 213 mg   Calcium: 152 mg

Cherry-Cheese Mousse

Yield: 6 servings

4 ounces block-style light (Neufchâtel) cream cheese, softened to
   room temperature
Sugar substitute equal to ¼ cup sugar
½ cup nonfat or light sour cream
20-ounce can no-added-sugar or light (reduced-sugar) cherry
   pie-filling
2 cups nonfat or light whipped topping

1. Place the cream cheese and sugar substitute in a large bowl, and beat with an electric mixer until smooth. Add the sour cream and beat to mix well. Fold in first the pie filling and then the whipped topping.
2. Divide the dessert between six 8-ounce wine glasses. Cover and refrigerate for at least 2 hours before serving.

Nutritional Facts (per ¾-cup serving)

Calories: 147   Carbohydrates: 20 g   Cholesterol: 13 mg   Fat: 4.9 g   Saturated Fat: 2.7 g   Fiber: 1.1 g   Protein: 3.2 g   Sodium: 120 mg   Calcium: 37 mg

Creamy Chocolate Custard

Yield: 5 servings

12-ounce can evaporated nonfat or low-fat milk
3 tablespoons light brown sugar
⅓ cup chopped dark chocolate or semi-sweet chocolate chips

¾ cup fat-free egg substitute
1 teaspoon vanilla extract

1. Preheat the oven to 325 degrees.
2. Place the milk, brown sugar, and chocolate in a 2-quart microwave-safe bowl. Microwave at high power for several minutes, whisking after each minute, or until the chocolate is completely melted.
3. Stir about ½ cup of the hot milk mixture into the egg substitute, then whisk the egg substitute mixture into the milk mixture. Whisk in the vanilla extract.
4. Coat five 6-ounce custard cups with cooking spray and divide the custard mixture among the cups. Arrange the custard cups in a large baking pan and fill the pan with 1 inch of hot tap water.
5. Bake uncovered for 25 to 30 minutes or until a sharp knife inserted near the center of the custards comes out clean. Remove the custards from the pan and let cool for 1 hour at room temperature. Cover and chill until ready to serve.
6. To serve, loosen the edges with a sharp knife and invert each custard onto a dessert plate. If desired, garnish with fresh raspberries or chopped walnuts and a drizzle of light chocolate syrup.

Nutritional Facts (per serving)
Calories: 162   Carbohydrates: 24 g   Cholesterol: 3 mg   Fat: 3.5 g   Saturated Fat: 2.1 g   Fiber: 0.7 g   Protein: 10 g   Sodium: 167 mg   Calcium: 245 mg

Chocolate Clusters

Yield: 18 pieces

6 ounces semi-sweet or bittersweet chocolate, coarsely chopped
1½ cups nuts (use slivered or coarsely chopped almonds; pecan or
   walnut halves; coarsely chopped macadamia nuts; or roasted
   unsalted cashews or peanuts)

1. Place the chocolate in a 1½-quart microwave-safe bowl and microwave at high power for 3 minutes, stirring after every minute, until the chocolate is melted. Stir in the nuts, and drop heaping teaspoonfuls of the mixture onto

a large baking sheet lined with waxed paper. Flatten slightly with the tip of a spoon.

2. Place baking sheet in the refrigerator for at least one hour or until the clusters are no longer sticky to the touch. Arrange the clusters in a single layer in an airtight container and cover until ready to serve.

Nutritional Facts (per piece)

*Calories: 91   Carbohydrate: 6 g   Cholesterol: 0 mg   Fat: 7.8 g   Saturated Fat: 2.4 g
Fiber: 1.2 g   Protein: 2.4 g   Sodium: 3 mg   Calcium: 25 mg*

Stuffed Strawberries

Yield: 24 strawberries

24 medium fresh strawberries, rinsed and patted dry
8 ounces reduced-fat (Neufchâtel) cream cheese
3 tablespoons sugar substitute or sugar
2 tablespoons finely chopped hazelnuts or almonds

1. Cut a thin slice off the stem end of each strawberry so they will sit upright without falling over. Starting at the pointed end of the berry, cut a slit down the middle of each berry almost to the stem end, taking care not to cut the berry in half.
2. Beat the cream cheese and sugar substitute or sugar with an electric mixer until smooth. Transfer the filling to a pastry bag fitted with a star tip. Pull each berry apart just enough to pipe about 1½ teaspoons into the centers. (If you don't have a pastry bag, place the cheese mixture in a small plastic zip-type bag, snip a small piece from a bottom corner of the bag, and use that to fill the berries. Or simply spoon some of the filling into each berry.)
3. Stand the berries upright and sprinkle each one with ¼ teaspoon of the nuts. Serve immediately, or cover and refrigerate for 1 to 3 hours before serving.

Nutritional Facts (per strawberry)

*Calories: 33   Carbohydrates: 1.6 g   Cholesterol: 7 mg   Fat: 2.4 g   Saturated Fat:
1.4 g   Fiber: 0.5 g   Protein: 1.2 g   Sodium: 40 mg   Calcium: 10 mg*

Spiced Summer Fruits

Yield: 5 servings

2 cups chilled diced fresh mangos

2 cups chilled fresh blueberries, rinsed and patted dry

2 tablespoons frozen orange juice concentrate, thawed

2 tablespoons honey

⅛ to ¼ teaspoon ground ginger

3 tablespoons sliced almonds

1. Place the mangos and blueberries in a medium bowl and toss to mix well. Divide the mixture between five 8-ounce dessert dishes.

2. Place the juice concentrate, honey, and ginger in a small bowl, and stir to mix well. Drizzle a quarter of the mixture over each dish of fruit. Serve immediately, topping each serving with a sprinkling of almonds.

Nutritional Facts (per serving)

Calories: 135   Carbohydrates: 29 g   Cholesterol: 0 mg   Fat: 2.4 g   Saturated Fat: 0.2 g   Fiber: 3.2 g   Protein: 1.8 g   Sodium: 6 mg   Calcium: 21 mg

Ricotta-Stuffed Peaches

Yield: 4 servings

2 large peaches (8 ounces each)

¼ cup plus 2 tablespoons part skim ricotta cheese or soft curd farmer's cheese

1 tablespoon plus 1 teaspoon honey

2 tablespoons chopped toasted pecans or sliced toasted almonds (page 240)

1. Cut the peaches in half and remove the pits. Cut a thin slice off the bottom of each peach half so it will sit upright.

2. Place a peach half in each of 4 dessert dishes. Mound 1½ tablespoons of the cheese in the center of each peach half and drizzle with a teaspoon of

honey. Top each serving with a sprinkling of the pecans or almonds. Serve immediately.

Nutritional Facts (per serving)

Calories: 128   Carbohydrates: 19 g   Cholesterol: 7 mg   Fat: 4.6 g   Saturated Fat: 1.4 g   Fiber: 2.6 g   Protein: 4 g   Sodium: 29 mg   Calcium: 71 mg

Baked Brandied Peaches

Yield: 5 servings

5 cups sliced fresh peeled peaches
2 tablespoons light brown sugar
Sugar substitute equal to 2 tablespoons sugar
2 to 3 tablespoons brandy

1. Preheat the oven to 425 degrees.
2. Coat a 9-by-13-inch pan with nonstick cooking spray and spread the peaches in the pan. Combine the brown sugar and sugar substitute, sprinkle over the peaches, and drizzle with the brandy.
3. Bake uncovered for 8 minutes, stir the mixture, and bake for an additional 4 minutes, or until the peaches are tender. Serve warm. If desired, serve over a scoop of light vanilla ice cream.

Nutritional Facts (per ½-cup serving)

Calories: 106   Carbohydrate: 24 g   Cholesterol: 0 mg   Fat: 0.1 g   Saturated Fat: 0 g Fiber: 3.4 g   Protein: 1.2 g   Sodium: 2 mg   Calcium: 13 mg

Citrus-Spiked Berries

Yield: 5 servings

2 cups fresh strawberries, rinsed, patted dry, and quartered
1 cup fresh raspberries
1 cup fresh blackberries or blueberries
2 tablespoons Grand Marnier or orange liqueur

2 tablespoons sugar

1 tablespoon orange juice concentrate

1. Place the fruits in a medium bowl. Combine the liqueur, sugar, and juice concentrate in a small bowl and stir to mix well.
2. Pour the liqueur mixture over the berries and toss to mix well. Let the mixture sit at room temperature for 30 minutes before serving.

Nutritional Facts (per serving)

Calories: 95   Carbohydrate: 20 g   Cholesterol: 0 mg   Fat: 0.5 g   Saturated Fat: 0 g
Fiber: 4.7 g   Protein: 0.9 g   Sodium: 1 mg   Calcium: 25 mg

Pears with Raspberry Sauce

Yield: 6 servings

RASPBERRY SAUCE
3⅓ cups fresh raspberries
Sugar substitute equal to 3 tablespoons sugar
1 tablespoon sugar
1 teaspoon lemon juice

2 cans (15 ounces each) pear halves packed in juice, chilled and
   drained
¼ cup sliced toasted almonds (page 240) or shaved dark chocolate

1. To make the sauce, place 2 cups of the raspberries in a blender or food processor. Add the sugar substitute, sugar, lemon juice, and 1½ tablespoons of the juice from the canned pears, and purée until smooth. Pour the mixture into a wire strainer and, using the back of a spoon, push the mixture through the strainer and into a bowl. Discard the seeds. Set the sauce aside.
2. Using a sharp knife, slice each pear half lengthwise toward the narrow end without cutting completely to the end, and open each pear half into a fan shape.
3. Place 2 tablespoons of the raspberry sauce on each of 6 dessert plates. Top

the sauce on each plate with 2 pear fans and garnish with some of the remaining fresh raspberries, and almonds, or chocolate. Serve immediately.

Nutritional Facts (per serving)

Calories: 102   Carbohydrate: 20 g   Cholesterol: 0 mg   Fat: 2.5 g   Saturated Fat: .   0.2 g   Fiber: 4 g   Protein: 1.7 g   Sodium: 9 mg   Calcium: 27 mg

Frozen Banana Dream Pie

Yield: 10 servings

12 sugar-free cream-filled chocolate sandwich cookies,
   coarsely crushed
⅓ cup peanut butter
Sugar substitute equal to 2 tablespoons sugar
⅓ cup nonfat or low-fat milk
1 cup sliced bananas
4 cups low-fat or light no-added-sugar vanilla ice cream,
   slightly softened
3 tablespoons light (reduced-sugar) chocolate syrup

1. Spread the cookies evenly over the bottom of a 9-inch springform pan. Place the peanut butter and sugar substitute in a medium bowl and slowly add the milk, whisking until smooth. Drizzle the mixture over the cookies and then top with the banana slices.
2. Spoon the ice cream evenly over the layers. Cover the pan and freeze for 8 hours or until firm.
3. When ready to serve, remove the dessert from the freezer and let sit for 10 to 15 minutes at room temperature before slicing. Drizzle each piece with some of the chocolate syrup just before serving.

Nutritional Facts (per serving)

Calories: 205   Carbohydrate: 30 g   Cholesterol: 8 mg   Fat: 8.3 g   Saturated Fat: 2 g   Fiber: 2 g   Protein: 6 g   Sodium: 143 mg   Calcium: 103 mg

Ice Cream with Apricot-Brandy Sauce

Yield: 4 servings

SAUCE

1 cup chopped canned (drained) apricot halves

1 tablespoon apricot brandy

Sugar substitute equal to 1½ tablespoons sugar

2 cups low-fat or light no-added-sugar vanilla ice cream

¼ cup toasted sliced almonds or chopped toasted pecans
  (page 240)

1. To make the sauce, place the apricots, brandy, and sugar substitute in a blender or food processor and process until smooth. Set aside.
2. To assemble the desserts, place a ½-cup scoop of ice cream in each of 4 dessert dishes. Top the ice cream in each dish with a quarter of the sauce, then sprinkle with a quarter of the almonds or pecans. Serve immediately.

Nutritional Facts (per serving)

Calories: 165   Carbohydrate: 23 g   Cholesterol: 10 mg   Fat: 5.3 g   Saturated Fat: 1.3 g   Fiber: 2.3 g   Protein: 4.8 g   Sodium: 63 mg   Calcium: 119 mg

Really Raspberry Sundaes

Yield: 4 servings

SAUCE

2 cups frozen unsweetened raspberries, thawed

Sugar substitute equal to 2 to 3 tablespoons sugar

2 tablespoons raspberry liqueur

2 cups low-fat or light no-added-sugar vanilla ice cream

¼ cup chopped walnuts

1. To make the sauce, place the berries in a small wire strainer and use the back of a spoon to force the berries through the strainer and into a bowl. Con-

Selecting the Best Ice Cream

Countless brands of "sugar-free" and "no-added-sugar" brands of ice cream are now available to choose from. These products are typically sweetened with a combination of sugar alcohols and artificial sweeteners, and have 25 to 50 percent fewer carbs than regular ice cream. The caveat is many of these products are loaded with saturated fat and save you few or no calories.

What should you look for when buying ice cream? First, go for a low-fat or light brand, as this will limit your intake of artery-clogging saturated fat. Next, consider calories and carbohydrates and choose a brand that is moderate in both. But above all, choose a brand that you really *enjoy* eating. As with many other foods, ultra-low-carb versions may be a poor substitute for the real thing, leaving you unsatisfied and longing for something better. Finally, realize that no ice cream is totally sugar-free because some sugar (lactose) is naturally present in the milk that ice cream is made from.

tinue to mash the berries and force them through the strainer until only the seeds remain in the strainer. Discard the seeds and add the sugar substitute and liqueur to the berry pulp, and stir to mix.

2. To assemble the desserts, place a ½-cup scoop of ice cream in each of 4 dessert dishes. Top the ice cream in each dish with a quarter of the sauce, then sprinkle with a quarter of the walnuts. Serve immediately.

Nutritional Facts (per serving)

Calories: 191   Carbohydrate: 25 g   Cholesterol: 10 mg   Fat: 6.5 g   Saturated Fat: 1.3 g   Fiber: 1.8 g   Protein: 5 g   Sodium: 60 mg   Calcium: 109 mg

Light Root-Beer Float

Yield: 1 serving

¾ cup low-fat or light no-added-sugar vanilla ice cream
¾ cup sugar-free root beer

1. Place the ice cream in a 12-ounce glass. Pour the root beer over the ice cream.
2. Stir to slightly blend the ice cream and soda. Serve immediately.

Nutritional Facts (per serving)

*Calories: 150   Carbohydrate: 25 g   Cholesterol: 15 mg   Fat: 3 g   Saturated Fat: 1.5 g
Fiber: 1.5 g   Protein: 4.5 g   Sodium: 110 mg   Calcium: 150 mg*

Selected References

1.   Agus MSD et al. Dietary composition and physiologic adaptations to energy restriction. *American Journal of Clinical Nutrition* 2000;71:901–7.

2.   Baba NH et al. High protein vs. high carbohydrate hypoenergetic diet for the treatment of obese hyperinsulinemic subjects. *International Journal of Obesity and Related Metabolic Disorders* 1999;11:1202–6.

3.   Bouche C et al. Five-week, low-glycemic index diet decreases total fat mass and improves plasma lipid profile in moderately overweight nondiabetic men. *Diabetes Care* 2002; 25:822–28.

4.   Brehm BJ et al. A randomized trial comparing a very low carbohydrate diet and a calorie-restricted low fat diet on body weight and cardiovascular risk factors in healthy women. *Journal of Clinical Endocrinology and Metabolism* 2003;88:1617–23.

5.   Carruth BR and Skinner JD. The role of dietary calcium and other nutrients in moderation of body fat in preschool children. *International Journal of Obesity and Related Metabolic Disorders*. 2001;25;559–66.

6.   Dumesnil JG et al. Effect of a low glycemic index, low-fat, high-protein diet on the atherogenic metabolic risk profile of abdominally obese men. *British Journal of Nutrition* 2001;86:557–68.

7.   Eaton SB and Eaton SB III. Paleolithic vs. modern diets—selected pathophysiological implications. *European Journal of Nutrition* 2000;39(2):67–70.

8.   Eaton SB et al. Evolutionary health promotion: a consideration of common counterarguments. *Preventive Medicine* 2002;35(4):415–18.

9.   Eaton SB et al. Paleolithic nutrition revisited: a twelve-year retrospective on its nature and implications. *European Journal of Clinical Nutrition*. 1997;51:207–16.

10.   Ebbeling CB et al. A reduced-glycemic load diet in the treatment of adolescent obesity. *Archives of Pediatric and Adolescent Medicine* 2003;157:773–79.

11.   Ford ES et al. Prevalence of the metabolic syndrome among U.S. adults. *Journal of the American Medical Association* 2002;287:356–59.

12. Foster GD et al. A randomized trial of a low-carbohydrate diet for obesity. *New England Journal of Medicine* 2003;348:2082–90.

13. Giannini S et al. Acute effects of moderate dietary protein restriction in patients with idiopathic hypercalcuria and calcium nephrolithiasis. *American Journal of Clinical Nutrition* 1999;69:267–71.

14. Golay A et al. Weight loss with low or high carbohydrate diet? *International Journal of Obesity* 1996;20:1067–72.

15. Heaney RP et al. Calcium and weight: clinical studies. *Journal of the American College of Nutrition* 2002;21(2):152S–55S.

16. Hu FB et al. Television watching and other sedentary behaviors in relation to risk of obesity and type 2 diabetes mellitus in women. *Journal of the American Medical Association* 2003;289(14):1785–91.

17. Hu FB et al. Dietary protein and risk of ischemic heart disease in women. *American Journal of Clinical Nutrition* 1999;70:221–27.

18. Jiang R et al. Nut and peanut butter consumption and risk of type 2 diabetes in women. *Journal of the American Medical Association* 2002;288(20):2554–60.

19. Johnston CS et al. Postprandial thermogenesis is increased 100% on a high-protein, low-fat diet versus a high-carbohydrate, low-fat diet in healthy young women. *Journal of the American College of Nutrition* 2002;21(1):55–61.

20. Knight EL et al. The impact of protein intake on renal function decline in women with normal renal function or mild renal insufficiency. *Annals of Internal Medicine* 2003; 138(6):460–67.

21. Kris-Etherton PM et al. AHA Scientific Statement: Fish consumption, fish oil, omega-3 fatty acids, and cardiovascular disease. *Circulation* 2002;106:2747–57.

22. Layman DK et al. A reduced ratio of dietary carbohydrate to protein improves body composition and blood lipid profiles during weight loss in adult women. *Journal of Nutrition* 2003;133:411–17.

23. Lean ME et al. Weight loss with high and low carbohydrate 1200 kcal diets in free living women. *European Journal of Clinical Nutrition* 1997;51(4): 243–48.

24. Ludwig DS et al. High glycemic index foods, overeating, and obesity. *Pediatrics* 1999;103(3):261–66.

25. McNutt K. What clients need to know about sugar replacers. *Journal of the American Dietetic Association* 2000;100(4):466–69.

26. Miller SL and Wolfe RR. Physical exercise as a modulator of adaptation to low and high carbohydrate and low and high fat intakes. *European Journal of Clinical Nutrition* 1999; 53(Suppl 1):S112–19.

27. Munger RG et al. Prospective study of dietary protein intake and risk of hip fracture in postmenopausal women. *American Journal of Clinical Nutrition* 1999;69:147–52.

28. National Institutes of Health, National Heart Lung, and Blood Institute. *Third Report of the National Cholesterol Education Program Expert Panel on Detection, Evaluation, and Treatment of High Blood Cholesterol in Adults (Adult Treatment Panel III)*. NIH Publication 02-5215; September 2002. Accessed online 8/6/03 at http://www.nhlbi.nih.gov/guidelines/cholesterol/atp3full.pdf.

29. Painter JE et al. How visibility and convenience influence candy consumption. *Appetite*. 2002 Jun;38(3):237–38.

30. Parker B et al. Effect of a high-protein, high-monounsaturated fat weight loss diet on glycemic control and lipid levels in type 2 diabetes. *Diabetes Care* 2002;25:425–30.

31. Pawlak DB et al. High glycemic index starch promotes hypersecretion of insulin and higher body fat in rats without affecting insulin sensitivity. *Journal of Nutrition* 2001;131:99–104.

32. Periera MA et al. Effect of whole grains on insulin sensitivity in overweight hyper-insulinemic adults. *American Journal of Clinical Nutrition* 2002;75:848–55.

33. Periera MA et al. Dairy consumption, obesity, and the insulin resistance syndrome in young adults. *Journal of the American Medical Association* 2002;287;2081–89.

34. Piatti PM et al. Hypocaloric high-protein diet improves glucose oxidation and spares lean body mass: comparison to hypocaloric high-carbohydrate diet. *Metabolism* 1994; 43(12):1481–87.

35. Promislow JHE et al. Protein consumption and bone mineral density in the elderly. *American Journal of Epidemiology* 2002;155(7):636–44.

36. Reddy ST et al. Effect of low-carbohydrate high-protein diets on acid-base balance, stone-forming propensity, and calcium metabolism. *American Journal of Kidney Diseases* 2002;40(2):265–74.

37. Roughead ZK et al. Controlled high meat diets do not affect calcium retention or indices of bone status in healthy postmenopausal women. *Journal of Nutrition* 2003;133: 1020–26.

38. Sabate J. Nut consumption and body weight. *American Journal of Clinical Nutrition* 2003. 78(3):647S–50S.

39. Samaha FF et al. A low-carbohydrate as compared with a low-fat diet in severe obesity. *New England Journal of Medicine* 2003;348:2074–81.

40. Sharman MJ et al. A ketogenic diet favorably affects serum biomarkers for cardiovascular disease in normal-weight men. *Journal of Nutrition* 2002;132:1879–85.

41. Skov AR et al. Effect of protein intake on bone mineralization during weight loss: a 6-month trial. *Obesity Research* 2002;10(6):432–38.

42. Skov AR et al. Randomized trial on protein vs. carbohydrate in ad libitum fat reduced diet for the treatment of obesity. *International Journal of Obesity and Related Metabolic Disorders* 1999;23(5):528–36.

43. Skov AR et al. Changes in renal function during weight loss by high vs. low-protein low-fat diets in overweight subjects. *International Journal of Obesity and Related Metabolic Disorders* 1999;23(11):1170–7.

44. Spieth LE et al. A low-glycemic index diet in the treatment of pediatric obesity. *Archives of Pediatric and Adolescent Medicine* 2000;154:947–51.

45. Westman EC et al. Effect of 6-month adherence to a very low carbohydrate diet program. *American Journal of Medicine* 2002;113:30–36.

46. Wolfe BMJ and Piche LA. Replacement of carbohydrate by protein in a conventional-fat diet reduces cholesterol and triglycerides concentrations in healthy normolipidemic subjects. *Clinical Investigations in Medicine* 1999;22(4):140–48.

47. Yanovski S. Sugar and fat: cravings and aversions. *Journal of Nutrition* 2003;133: 835S–37S.

48. Yunsheng M et al. Association between eating patterns and obesity in a free-living U.S. adult population. *American Journal of Epidemiology* 2003. 158:85–92.

49. Zemel MB et al. Dairy (yogurt) augments fat loss and reduces central adiposity during energy restriction in obese subjects. *FASEB* 2003;17(5):A1088.

50. Zemel MB. Role of dietary calcium and dairy products in modulating adiposity. *Lipids* 2003;38(2):139–46.

Index

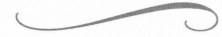